MW00510775

# TODDLER DISCIPLINE FOR BUSY PARENTS

Written By

## Jennifer Siegel

# Table of Contents

# INTRODUCTION

*Thank you for purchasing this book!*

Connection or secure attachment is one of the significant biological needs of humans. It is no surprise that children have a strong passion for their parents. Parents provide their needs for optimal development and survival. It is necessary to put your love into action, meet your child's needs, pay attention, respect his views, and instill loving guidance or discipline to establish a strong connection. Without secure attachment or when conditions are not satisfied, the outcomes are retardation of growth and occurrences of destructive behaviors.

During the toddler stage, your child wants independence but still afraid to be separated from you. He starts to realize that he has strong feelings, but does not know how to express or control them. Moreover, the child discovers that he has a power that can make others give him what he needs and will test it now and then. All these things are opportunities for parents to nurture their connection to their toddlers. The relationship is also the vital key that makes the child willing to follow the rules you set with willingness and cooperation.

# Explain Yourself

At 24 months and up, toddlers are beginning to understand what is right and what is not. Unfortunately, it is also the stage where sharing is difficult for the child, not wanting to share your attention, time, or even toys. And what complicates the matter more is he begins to snatch everything he likes. The good news is that toddlers can comprehend the cause and effect and follow the simple instructions, so you can try saying, "We don't grab the toys of others" and give him his toys.

This is why you must explain to your child the reason behind your rule or instruction. It helps him see and decide which is the better option or behavior. Inform the child about your expectations, precisely the action you want him to demonstrate.

For example, you see your kid with a crayon and going closer to the wall. Refrain from yanking the crayon and yelling "no," instead hug him gently to divert his attention. You can also give him a piece of paper, explaining that coloring is nice, but it should not be done on the walls.

As much as possible, avoid telling him what not to do or stopping his attempt by saying, "no." According to child experts, toddlers who hear many "no" everyday display more deficient language skills. It also becomes ineffective when overused, prompting the kid to ignore it or shriek the minute he hears it from the parent.

*Enjoy your reading!*

# Positive Parenting

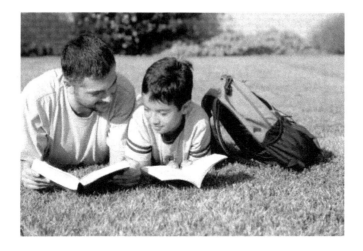

Positive parenting is defined as a style of parenting that emphasizes mutual respect. It is also referred to as gentle guidance, affectionate guidance, or loving guidance that places or keeps the child on the correct path. It uses positive discipline, instructions, and reinforcements geared at training the child to become a self-disciplined, responsible, and confident person. It involves teaching the child the who, where, when, what, and why of every situation. Its primary goal is to develop a deeply-committed, open, healthy, and strong relationship between the child and the parent.

It is an approach that helps children feel connected, connected, capable, and cooperative. It is not just about letting go of punishment or being permissive. Positive parenting is choosing to become actively involved in connecting and supporting their optimum growth and development. Generally speaking, positive parenting nurtures the child's self-esteem, sense of mastery, ability to interact, and belief in the future by living a productive, open, and healthy life.

# Vital Elements Of Positive Parenting

- Imagine or understand the point of view of the child during challenging times.

- Provide consistent and age-appropriate rules, limits, and expectations.

- Respond with sensitivity and interest to the cues that the child displays.

- Recognize the child's abilities, strengths, and capabilities to learn and then celebrate them to reinforce the development.

- Enjoy moments of connection.

- Work to attain a balanced time for child needs and parental needs.

- Understand that missteps are part of rearing a child, and sometimes, parenting can be stressful.

- Learn how to regulate your behaviors and emotions before responding to your child.

- Seek support, help, and parenting information if necessary.

Studies show that the child's experiences in his first three years of life are influenced by the quality of caring that he receives from his parents—the efforts to nurture, support, and raise him set his path to success and happiness. His young brain is recording and assimilating everything, processing them as truth and proper. Your habits become new habits.

# Effects of Positive Parenting

Positive parenting encourages children to respond to gentle guidance, improving their behavior, and developing self-discipline. In the absence of threats and punishments, children discover their strengths, power, and capabilities. It teaches children to accept their flaws or weaknesses and work to improve them.

It offers many benefits which include:

A. Maintaining quality parent-child relationship.

A fostering connection between you and your child is the foundation for developing good character traits, behavior, and confidence. Positive parenting is characterized by firm, loving guidance that builds a stronger connection and relationship. When you consider the long-term effects of positive parenting on your child, you know that you are on the right track.

The parental relationship is the most significant and influential connection that sets the bar for the child's cheerful disposition in life, success, and behavior. The strong bond fosters better decision-making, boosts self-esteem, encourage autonomy, and promote cooperation.

- Be involved. Enrich your relationship by connecting with your child using an age-appropriate approach. If your child is still a toddler, play with him, work on fun and creative projects, and teach him to read. If you have an adolescent child, challenge him in his favorite video game or sport. This technique will make him see you as an approachable parent.

- Emphasize on family time. A habit to eat dinner together or do something together during weekends. By establishing a regular family togetherness, you teach your child the importance of family as a unit.

- Set a one-on-one time for your child.

Spending quality time with your child is priceless. It helps you monitor his progress and development, making him feel your presence in every step of his journey as a person. Recognize his talents, strengths, and interests. Use the time to instill positive discipline by talking about situations that he considers problematic and finding ways to resolve the problems permanently. Build a meaningful and memorable bond by engaging in fun or educational activities.

- Get in touch with his academic and extracurricular activities. No matter how busy you are, making an effort to learn about his daily activities will make him feel loved and important. Ask about his friends at school, sit down with him when he is doing homework, help him check before the test, attend his school events, or invite his friends.

## B. Taking responsibility for actions

Become the model of accountability by being humble and honest to admit that you are wrong. Teach him the importance of saying sorry and being responsible for his action or reactions over matters that affect relationships.

Before you can effectively teach your kid about taking responsibility for his actions, it is necessary to recognize and understand the "why" that triggers his behavior. There is a reason why he misbehaves, not just to get into trouble or annoy you. As a parent, you have to find it out in ways that will not offend, hurt, or embarrass him.

•Respond, but do not react. Avoid overreacting and take a deep breath. Do not force him to apologize or become accountable immediately. Give time for both of you to calm down.

•Make it safe for him to come forward. Once everyone is calm, let him approach you and explain his behavior or admit the truth. Another option is to approach him and talk about what happened. If he admits his wrongdoing and apologizes, you need to acknowledge the effort, discuss how it can be prevented in the future, and enforce his action's corresponding consequence.

• Stick to your rules and limits. No matter how pitiful his pleadings or how sweet he becomes after his misbehavior, it is essential to be consistent with your discipline strategy. Don't give in if you want to convince him that you are serious about the rules.

• Talk about action or behavior, not the person. Instead of pointing out your child's flaw, focus your attention on his behavior, and find the reason behind it. Let him voice out his sentiments, feelings, and thoughts. Empathize with his struggles, listen to what he is telling you, read between the lines, and work together to find an appropriate solution that will prevent the action's recurrence.

C. Being respectful to others

One of the goals of positive discipline and positive parenting is fostering mutual respect. Respect is a two-way process. If you want to raise a respectful child, it is essential to model the behavior. Home is the first place where he learns about this fundamental virtue, so you need to teach respect as early as possible.

• Lead by example. Kids are very impressionable. They naturally mimic the habits of people who are around them while growing up and look up to them as role models. Start teaching your child the value of respect, living a respectful, and leading a loving and kind life.

• Use respect as a tool for him to get what he likes. In the adult world, people who show affection are most likely to get what they want. Teach this to your child by only giving the something he wants when he is respectful. He will soon realize that it is a quicker and smarter way rather than throwing a fit.

• Encourage activities that require cooperation and sharing. One example that teaches these virtues is a board game. Every player needs to respect the time that other players take to consider their moves.

•Be patient. Patience is a manifestation of respect. To teach it effectively, you should not display impatience when you are dealing with him. If he observes that you are not practicing what you are telling him, he will not imbibe the true essence of patience.

D. Knowing the difference between right and wrong.

Recent studies revealed that 19-21 months old babies could understand the sense of fairness or the right from the wrong. The quality of care that children experience in the early months of his life lays the foundation of a positive parent-child relationship. The first five years of their lives are crucial periods of moral, social, and emotional development. Their understanding of justice and fairness expands as they grow.

At ages 0 to 1, the infant learns right from wrong through experience. He feels that something is wrong when he is wet or hungry. If he is adequately attended and nurtured, he feels good and right. By the time he is 1-year old, he can communicate his feelings through actions and preferences, initiate contact, imitate, and develop a deeper understanding of what is right to do and what is not.

At ages 1-3, the toddler learns to understand the concept of rules. He responds and stops his attempt if you tell him not to do something. However, sometimes, he cannot resist acting impulsively, like grabbing a toy from another child. At this period, he still cannot truly distinguish the right and wrong acts. The child relies on you or other pictures of authority to define them for him.

At ages 4-5, the preschooler child begins to develop his ideas of what is right and wrong based on what he sees and learns from the family. As his social exposure and interactions increase, the child's moral intelligence grows too. He becomes more aware of acceptable behavior and begins to develop a stronger sense of justice. At this stage, you need to be more vigilant and consistent with your reminders.

•Initiate discussions about ethical situations and encourage your child to talk about his feelings. It leads to the development of values and ethical behaviors that will guide him in his lifetime.

•Let him understand that people have different feelings and thoughts. This will develop his capacity to observe and respect other people's feelings, learning to respond with concern and care.

•Help your child understand his feelings. Make him realize that emotions are not wrong or right, but how he acts or reacts makes a big difference.

•Regularly discuss with your child your decisions or behaviors in the context of right and wrong.

E. Making good and wise decisions.

Decision making is a vital skill that your child needs to develop to become successful in all aspects of his life, especially when he becomes an adult. The choices and decisions he makes dictate the path and direction of his adult life. Thus, the importance of teaching your child how to make wise decisions.

It is necessary to teach him as early as possible because once he goes out to start interacting with the outside world, external influences will attempt to steal the decision-making from him. Most children who are good at decision making become victims because the popular culture easily sways them.

F. Being honest, trustworthy, and loyal.

Before you can effectively discipline your child, it is essential to affirm or reaffirm your connection by being honest with your feelings.

•If you want him to study, tell him how proud you are for the high score during the last examination.
• If you are nervous about how he runs across the parking lot without looking first on both sides, tell it to him.

When you impart your feelings, he is more likely to follow your wishes, creating a life-lasting pattern of making him anticipate or be concerned with others' feelings before acting.

# Positive Communication

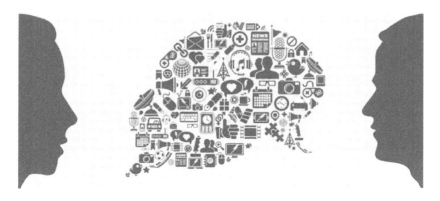

When my daughter wants to share information, she often asks, "Can I tell you something?" It's one of my favorite habits because I get to respond, "You can always tell me anything." Whether she's telling me about her joys and fears, how she's a part cheetah and part vampire, or plans for her birthday party, my intention is the same: to let her know that I am always there for her.

Communication is a top priority in our house. We tell our daughter we will always love her, no matter what. We tell her when we are getting frustrated. We talk about everything. I tell her she can ask me any question; I won't always have the answer, but she and I can find it together. All of this promotes a feeling of security and connection.

But this makes it sound easy. Real communication isn't always accessible or natural. It takes work and practice because what's easy is getting caught up in thoughts or distracted by automatic judgments or other things.

# Intention And Connection

Our choices are a vital foundation for good communication. Setting the intention to care first and foremost, to be open to what the other person is sharing and experiencing, and to be curious but nonjudgmental allows for real listening and connecting. We often come into a conversation with a specific, narrow agenda or distracted by other things, which tends to close us to a real exchange.

As with any other skill, good communication takes practice. This doesn't mean rehearsing what you're going to say but practicing noticing your intentions as you begin a conversation and working to be present, mindfully, and judgmental. You can do this with your children and your partner, co-workers, friends, or other family members. Notice if you've decided how the conversation is going to go before you start. Inhale before you speak and, while the other person is saying, see if you can be open to what this person might offer (even if you disagree). Notice what it's like to be curious and care about connecting with this person, in whatever way is appropriate. The practice is vital because we are trying to build new habits, and when we are tired or stressed, we tend to fall back into our old, not always helpful patterns.

With positive parenting, we want to prioritize connection first and foremost. This isn't just about getting children to do something or having our say. How we say something often matters more than what we say. If we come to a conversation agitated, stressed, and distracted, our children will feel and feed off that and will be less likely to feel connected to us. If we are focused on being present with kindness and curiosity, they will feel heard.

Not every conversation needs to be an in-depth, life-changing discussion. You could have meaningful conversations when you pick the kids up from school or when you are asking them if they brushed their teeth. It's about choosing to connect first.

## <u>Listening</u>

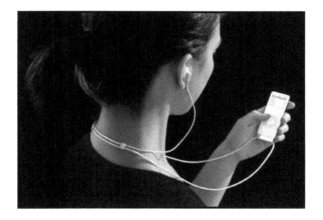

Just like us, children want to be heard. And although we want to be good listeners, life often gets in the way. Think about how often your child gets interrupted. It's probably a lot. When we interrupt them, we give them the message that what they have to say isn't necessary. Admittedly, your four-year-old's treatise on dinosaurs might not be the most scintillating thing you've heard. But again, this is about the long term. We inform them that we care, and their voices matter.

This isn't to say that you can never interrupt. If your child is anything like mine, you might have to interrupt; otherwise, you won't get a word in at all. We want to be clear about the intention to listen and be present for what they have to say.

Likewise, think about how many times we say things like, "You can't possibly be hungry; you just ate," or "Why are you so tired? You had a good night's sleep," or "But you love your gymnastics class." It's natural to react this way, but once we do so, we've not only closed ourselves off to hearing what's going on, but we might also be leading our children to doubt that we trust them, making it less likely that they will continue to be open and honest with us about how they are feeling.

To foster trust, build more connections, and promote our children's healthy development, it's essential to seek to understand their needs and their position. We need to listen openly and with the intention of closeness, without preparing a response in advance.

We just listen to what they say. It makes a more significant impact to be open to what they are feeling and going through and to let them know we care. When they say something that gets our blood boiling or makes us concerned, we have the opportunity to be aware of those reactions, to check our nervous systems, and then to communicate openly back to them: "I hear you saying that you want to ___. That makes me feel nervous. Can we talk about it some more?"

You might consider scheduling a monthly family meeting or event that lets everyone share openly. Conversations over the dishes are good, but it's useful to supplement them with time devoted to communicating. This also enables children to know there is always space for them to share. And yes, if you have older kids, this suggestion might engender serious eye-rolling, but that's mostly unavoidable at this point, so you might as well go for it anyway.

# Talking

It is helpful to have specific techniques for communicating. Our approach in this book is based on nonviolent communication (also known as compassionate communication). Pioneered by Marshall Rosenberg, it's an approach that offers specific strategies to build on the innate human capacities for compassion and empathy.

Generally, it's more supportive of expressing what's going on in terms of what you see and how it makes you feel rather than what the other person is doing or automatic reactions. "You are so frustrating" can shut down the conversation a lot faster than "I feel very frustrated right now."

This approach follows four main components, which both the speaker and the empathic listener use.

1. Observations: saying/receiving what you see, feel, hear, remember, imagine as objectively and nonjudgmentally as possible

2. Feelings: saying/accepting what you are feeling, expressing emotions

3. Needs: sharing/receiving empathically what needs are not being met

4. Requests: offering/hearing concrete ideas that would help meet your needs

We can use the ubiquitous "clean your room" argument to illustrate what this might look like.

**Scenario one:**

After a stressful day, you see your child's room. It's filthy. You immediately get angry. This is the millionth time this has happened. You begin yelling, "I've asked you a million times to clean your room. It's disgusting! I don't remember you listening. Why can't you do what I ask for once?"

Now, imagine the child's reaction. Most of us can understand the parent's perspective, but these statements are full of judgments, blaming, and personal criticism. The child will likely feel attacked and possibly lash out in retaliation, leading to more arguing and less connection (and less room cleaning). This method of communication is more about punishment and autopilot than discipline and conscious response.

**Scenario two:**

After a stressful day, you see your child's room. It's filthy. You immediately get angry. This is the millionth time this has happened. You want to start yelling. You stop yourself and take a breath (or a more extended break) to decide how to deal with this situation before responding with: "I see there are clothes all over the floor and the bed isn't made. I'm feeling frustrated. I've asked you to clean it many times. It seems you don't respect the rules of the house that are important to me. Can you please clean everything up before dinner?"

You can imagine the child's reaction here, too. Besides looking at you like you've grown a second head because you're weird, this will make them pause. You aren't attacking or blaming. You are presenting the situation so that everyone can relate to it, and you're allowing them to respond.

How you apply this will vary widely depending on the situation and the age of your children. Yet even with a toddler, you can say, "I see dirty hands. That can lead to germs. Let's go wash our hands together."

And of course, nothing is magic. Communicating more effectively does not mean your child's room will stay clean, that they will listen, or that all yelling will cease. It's helpful to practice compassionate communication, but this is still a child's room (or curfew, or homework, or any of the other challenges we face) that we are talking about: They are rites of passage and aren't going away any time soon. But even if your house stays messy, you've opened up the path to tremendous respect, trust, and listening through more open, compassionate communication.

# Conversation Traps

Most of us regularly fall into certain unhelpful traps in conversations. The goal here isn't to beat ourselves up about them but to do our best to see when we fall into these traps, forgive ourselves, and then choose an approach that promotes more give-and-take. Some common downsides:

•Blaming the other person or ourselves: Even if someone is at fault, we want to encourage taking responsibility rather than casting blame.

•Global judgments: It's better to stay specific than to make overarching statements about ourselves or others.

•Black-and-white statements: There's almost always an exception to the rule. "Always" and "never" reports cut off chances for growth and change and make others defensive.

•Unhelpful listening: This includes not listening at all but also rushing in to advise without being asked, offering pity rather than empathy, one-upping the other person with our own story, or when a conversation turns into an interrogation.

# <u>Other Helpful Communication Hints</u>

Use do statements instead of don'ts: "Hold the cup with two hands" is a lot easier to follow than "Don't spill." It's tough for anyone to comply with a "don't" statement because it's not clear what should be done instead. To support our children better, it's best to use positively framed ideas.

Talking to them directly: Parents often talk to their partners or other adults about the children rather than talking to them. Part of empowering our children means trusting their (age-appropriate) maturity and responsibility. Understanding their level (for little ones) is crucial.

Use fewer words: Parents tend to over-explain and lecture when merely pointing something out is more effective. "I see dirty clothes on the floor" has more impact than "Your clothes are on the floor again. I've told you a hundred times that you have to pick up your clothes. You need to take more responsibility for yourself, et al."

Ask questions: Instead of lecturing, which they tune out anyway, get them involved. Ask your children, "How can we solve this?"

# Behavior

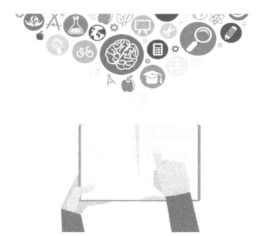

It's necessary for parents to bear in mind that kids are naturally good, and they have episodes of acting up due to specific reasons that they cannot voice out, especially when they are young and don't know how to process their emotions.

There are two factors behind your child's challenging behavior: the sense of not belonging (connection) and the sense of significance (contribution). When one or both basic needs are not satisfied, the children find a way to fulfill it, even if it requires adverse action. Dr. Dreikurs aptly put it by stating that "A misbehaving child is a discouraged child."

Calling the child as "bad" for doing something negative isn't healthy for their self-esteem. It usually starts when your kid continually misbehaves or throw tantrums, and you are exasperated. While trying to calm them, you lose control and label them as a "bad boy" or "bad girl" unintentionally. You can forgive yourself after that little slip and quote the famous cliché that you're just human, and humans make mistakes, but if you keep repeating it every time they do something wrong, it will be engraved in their mind and damage their self-worth.

Positive discipline aims to help parents learn to objectify the behavior and cut the "bad cycle." For example, instead of telling your child when they hit their younger sibling that "that's bad" or "you're such a bad boy," you may say, "it isn't okay to hit your brother when you are angry because they do not share their toy" and then let them understand the harm that might happen to their brother. When you objectify their behavior, you're teaching them the cause and effect. By directly addressing the "bad behavior" without using the term "bad," you're encouraging your child to make better choices and avoid hurting other people.

Show the child how to resolve the problem, instead of pointing out that what they did is wrong.

Redirecting your child's behavior requires more than saying, "Don't do that" or "No." It needs skills to teach them right from wrong using calm actions and words. For instance, you catch your child before they can hit their little brother, instead of saying "No hitting" or "Don't hit," tell them to "Ask their brother nicely if they want to borrow a toy." Other means to grab the toy, you're showing them that asking is more effective than hitting.

If they already hit their brother, it's a must to be creative with your response. One right way is enforcing a non-punitive time-out, which technically is about removing the child from the stimulus that triggers their behavior and allows them to calm down. You can cuddle them when they are agitated, let them play in their room, or ask them to sit with you and read a book. After their emotion subsides, start explaining (not lecturing) why their behavior is inappropriate. Please encourage your child to give other positive options that they believe will provide them with the result they want, without hurting anyone.

Be kind, yet firm when enforcing discipline. Show respect and empathy.

A child may insist that what they did was right, hence the importance of enforcing safety rules and consequences to prevent similar incidents in the future. Listen to their story as to why they did it and win half the battle by displaying empathy, but still impose the consequence of their action to learn from their mistakes. Kindness makes your child feel understood, lessening their resistance, and heightened emotions.

Look for the "why" behind this behavior, especially when you observe a pattern. Sometimes, hitting a sibling is a silent message that they are jealous of the attention you're giving to the younger child. Whatever the cause, resolve the issue early to make your child feels secure and loved. Get to the bottom reason of the problem.

Offer choices, whenever possible.

Giving your child positive choices works like magic when disciplining them. An example is when you're trying to make them sleep, and they still want to watch TV, instead of getting angry, provide choices. "Do you like to go to bed now or in ten minutes? Ten minutes? Okay, ten minutes and then off to bed."

This approach is a win-win solution because they get to pick the option that is okay with them, and you're offering choices that are advantageous to you. By not forcing them to do something and letting them choose, you prevent power struggle. You allow them to take charge and show autonomy within your parameters. To successfully use this technique, provide palatably, but limited choices. Eliminate options that are not acceptable to you and honor what they select.

Use mistakes as learning opportunities for your child.

Use every misbehaving episode as a chance to learn invaluable life lessons. Often, the child misbehaves to achieve what they want or when they are bored. For instance, they throw and break toys when they do not like them anymore. Instead of scolding them, use the opportunity to teach them the idea of giving them to their friends, or donating them. If they are bored, provide other exciting activities. This will teach them the concept of displacement or finding ways to be productive and prevent their properties. By empowering them with alternatives, they will be adept at making wise choices, even if you are not with them.

Prevent the repeat of misbehavior by changing the scene.

The famous adage still works – "Prevention is better than cure" in positive discipline. If you notice that your child keeps repeating an act, find ways to prevent it from recurring or resolve the problem.

One significant reason that you need to look into consideration is a transition. Most children do not like sudden changes, even in the ordinary routine. For instance, your child hates brushing their teeth in the morning and would do anything not to do it. Naturally, you will be frustrated because of the daily ordeal of resistance, which they show by crying, whining, screaming, hitting, or kicking.

What happens? It shows that they aren't resisting the act of brushing teeth; they are against the transition from sleep to a busy day because it overwhelms them. So, the next time your child repeats their tantrums over something, get to the leading cause and allows a transition time. For example, instead of rushing them to get dressed, set a timer that lets them do what they want, including getting ready. Ask him- "Do you need 20 or 30 minutes to get ready?" By letting them decide, they become in-charge of the allotted time but know that they need to show up dressed up before the time is up.

Be well-defined and stable with your expectancies and boundaries.

Children always find ways to push beyond the limits or find loopholes to satisfy their whims. They will attempt to test the limits to see your reaction or challenge you to know what will happen. So, it's necessary to talk to your child about the boundaries you set and the things you expect from them. Explain the corresponding consequences when they violate limits or house rules.

It is also essential to be consistent and follow through (do what you say) because it shows that you're serious about discipline. By being consistent, you're teaching them self-discipline, self-control, and other valuable lessons in life that will come in handy when they become an adult. Discipline requires a consistent application to be useful. Over time, they will recognize that their behavior and actions lead to consequences that they despise.

Use questions, state facts, or single-word reminders, instead of demanding or ordering them to comply.

When your baby grows into a toddler, you need to find language to make them comply and cooperate. Using respectful words is essential to make them obey you without saying "Stop" and "No." Connecting with your little child required breaking down communication barriers since they are still developing their speech skill.

It's much better to say, "Please look to your left and right before crossing the street," instead of ordering, "Don't cross the street without looking on your right and left." The word "Don't" serves as the modifier that confuses a little child. Say, for example, even if you cry out, "Don't jump in the puddle," your 2-year old kid still jump in and wonder why you're annoyed.

Treat and talk to them like an adult. Instead of ordering them, use positive phrasing, open questions, single-word reminders, or facts.

Use, "Shall we get up now?" instead of "Time to get up!"

"Shall we put these away, so nobody trips over them?" instead of yelling, "Put them away!"

"Your face is covered with chocolate! What shall we do about it?" instead of "Wipe your face."

"Light" instead of "Turn off the light after using the toilet."

"Kind words, please." instead of "Don't speak like that."

"Water is wasting," instead of "You are wasting water."

"We need to look after your little brother.", instead of "Don't hit the baby!"

How can we solve this problem?

Be generous with reasons, background information, facts, and explanations, so your child will better comprehend why they aren't allowed to do something or why they need to do it.

Involve them in problem-solving by working together as a team to find a mutually agreeable solution.

Children behave better on their free will when they see parents as allies. By giving your child a voice and the opportunity to be heard, they become more cooperative. Brainstorm solutions together and allow them to provide suggestions on matters that ensure safety and well-being.

Allow your kid to face natural consequences.

There are two types of consequences-natural and made-up. The latter are those that you make to suit your needs and propel them to comply. Some experts say that made-up consequences are punishments in disguise.

Categorically, made-up consequences come in forms of immediate effects, fair results, and logical development.

Immediate consequences help you teach the child to realize that their behavior is tied up with a result. An example is losing their phone privileges for a week when you find out that they are lying about getting their homework done.

Fair consequences are those that are reasonable and not overly harsh. If you ground them or prevent them from using electronics for one month, your kid would not think it's fair, and you are doing an injustice. They will fight the consequence every step of the way and try to defy it when you aren't around.

Logical consequences benefit children with specific behavior problems. An example is disallowing them to play with their toys if they refuse to put them back on the shelf. By linking the consequence with the problem, you let your child see that their choice directly results.

Natural consequences are part of natural growth. When you allow your kid to make mistakes and experience the natural results that arise from their misbehavior, you're showing them that inappropriate actions can lead them into trouble or face immediate consequences beyond your control.

For example, they touch the hot pot and get their hand burned. The pain is the natural consequence, teaching them not to do it again.

# Self-Efficacy And Self-Confidence

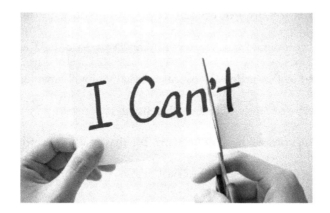

## <u>Self-Efficacy</u>

Some people work hard and strive for success, whereas on the other side, people just let their life pass without any specific aims or perspectives. People tend only to try things; they will believe they will be successful. For example, you work at a store, and they ask you to create a spreadsheet on the monthly sales. In your entire life, you have never created a spreadsheet. It doesn't mean that you should refuse the objective given; instead, you should strive and learn the spreadsheet to make a monthly sales report. If a person thinks that he can accomplish a task, the person will have a higher self-efficacy. On the other side, if the person feels that he cannot achieve the given mission, his self-efficacy level is low.

Several factors influence Self-efficacy:

- Performance Accomplishments: It means that how successful you have been in your past related to a specific task. Suppose you have applied for a course to learn PowerPoint. If you had no difficulty understanding the time, you would feel more confident in performing a task in the future related to PowerPoint. This means that you will have higher efficacy for this type of study. On the other hand, if you had issues in learning the course, you will hesitate to work for that field. Therefore, your efficacy level will be lower in the related field to that course.

In the children's case, your child would be more confident if he had easily accomplished the task before. Or else, the child would fear to try to do the homework again as he doesn't have trust in his abilities. This means that the child lacks self-efficacy. Parents should always boost their children for trying new things, and they should make sure that the child is happily engaged in the work. The first impression of anything on a children's brain will remain forever.

- Vicarious Experiences: It means to observe someone very similar to you. You will keep and implement the things in your life. For example, if your co-worker is working hard on a project and is trying to produce a great outcome, you will try to act similarly. Your efficacy level will increase, and you will have a very similar result. However, on the other hand, if the co-worker is struggling with a project and finding it hard to produce a result, your efficacy level will drop. You will also find it hard in that project.

In the case of children, they tend to follow their parents or their siblings. Sometimes we see children following the activities of their friends or siblings. If a random child is active in building a castle at a beach, your child will also make a higher efficacy. This means that the child has boosted his effectiveness by vicarious experiences.

- Verbal Persuasion: This is very similar to encouraging someone for a particular task. For example, if someone encourages you by saying, "You can do this.", the efficacy level will increase. However, on the other hand, if someone discourages you by saying, "This is too much for you." the efficacy level will decrease, and you will find it hard to complete that task.

The children are susceptible to verbal persuasion. If you keep on discouraging your child, this will have a disastrous impact on the child's brain development and growth. The entire personality will be ruined. They won't be productive in any part of life, and they would be scared of implanting new things. Moreover, they will not get curious about new learning activities. The discouragement would have a significant impact on their brain. Therefore, it is recommended to boost your children's courage and potential by continuously motivating them and encouraging them. Most importantly, they would be more productive if they hair praise for their effort than their abilities.

- Physiological States: It depends on the emotional state, mood, anxiety level, et al. If you are healthy, your efficacy is higher. If you are feeling low or sick, your effectiveness is more inferior.

In the case of children, it is linked with their health. If the child is healthy and active, he will have greater efficacy than a child feeling sluggish and sick all the time. The parents should keep great care of their children's health. Make sure that the immune system of the children is fully active and healthy. A slight distraction can bring massive harm to your child. Apart from this, keep interacting with your children. This will help you understand their problems and make a stronger bond with them. Their physiological state will improve with your little attention.

# Self-Confidence

It is the courage and ability to accept yourself or to believe in yourself. The definition is not sufficient itself, so let's give you an example. Suppose you are working in an organization, and you are a very hardworking employee. One day, your boss asks you to provide a presentation to the buyers. The buyers are essential for the organization, and the boss doesn't want to lose them. At this point, you have immense responsibility and pressure on your shoulders. Many of the people lose their skills, courage, abilities, and potential at this point. They lose their self-confidence and shiver with fear and anxiety. If you have self-confidence, you will have believed in yourself and your skills. You would have shown a more significant outcome than an average employee. Self-confidence provides the courage and ability to get your point of view approved. If you have self-confidence, you can achieve your goals.

Look around at those politicians; they dare to get their words approved in the assembly. From where do they get this potential and courage? It is all from self-confidence. To stand against the opposition, one must believe in oneself. If they don't believe in themselves, everyone will ignore their point of view. They will not be considered an essential part of the assembly. To be self-confident means you think the issues you are presenting and perusing people to follow it. Many of the great influencers, presenters, and speakers have self-confident. They know the way to keep their audience attracted to themselves. This is their skill, and they have trust in their mastery. For a more excellent example, refer to the motivational speakers. Look at the way they keep themselves attached to the audience. In no time, they create a bond with the viewers. Instead of fearing the people's reactions and views, they stand firm and deliver their thought with a great strategy. The strategy is nothing but self-confidence. Self-confidence is generated and build with experience.

The following factors influence self-confidence. The following factors are linked with the development of parent's self-confidence. The child learns from their parents, and the parents must develop self-confidence in themselves.

- Identify your negative thoughts: Your negative thinking creates a hindrance in your path to success. As we have learned in the belief system, the negative analysis is created by the conscious mind, and it harms the subconscious mind. Our self can control these negative thoughts. It just requires some motivation and uplifting. To boost and build your self-confidence, one must identify its negative thoughts and convert them into positive ones. Think more positive than negative; give complimentary analysis more space in your brain than negative reviews. The subconscious mind is like a warehouse, and filling it up with positivity will boost your self-confidence. Avoid unnecessary things that lower your self-confidence. Give time to yourself and mark things that disturb your peaceful mind. Filter them out, and you will observe the happiness in your life.

- Maintain a positive support network: If people keep on discouraging you, you will have low self-confidence. Your social pressure and fear will increase, and you will not interact much with the outer world. Let's take an example; you are a child whose parents keeps on discouraging their child by saying that the child is not capable and is weak. Even though the child is all good and perfect, he will feel sad and have lower self-confidence. This is just a small example related to motivation. If someone motivates you, you perform better. However, if someone continuously disturbs you and discourage you, the person will think negative of himself and will remain in depression. It is recommended to keep a positive support network. Stay in people that help you in your difficult time and stand beside you whenever you need any help. "A person is known by the company he keeps."

- Identify your talents and make a productive lifestyle: Keep yourself involved in your habits and interests. Permit yourself in taking pride in them. Express yourself through different hidden talents of yours. You will feel unique and accomplished. A greater probability of finding a compatible friend in your field of interest. Believe in yourself and start taking pride in yourself. For example, if a person loves singing and music, he will keep himself involved in his free time activities. He will have no time to think about the negativity around him. Interestingly, he can earn from his interests. This will make him more confident and will make him more relaxed in a hectic life. Moreover, accept the compliments gracefully. If you have a lower self-confidence level, you will find it hard to get a compliment from somebody. You will think that the person is either lying or mistaken.

- Stop comparing yourself with others: This is the biggest hindrance in the path to self-confidence. In this world, nobody is equal. Everyone has its potential, stamina, thinking, capabilities, strategies, et al. Don't make your life as your best friend's life. Think differently and make life as you desire than the desire of the people around you. Try to stand aside from the crowd as it requires self-confidence to be different.

- Learn from your mistakes: This is the essential tip in boosting your self-confidence. The ego destroys the personality of the people. Don't let your inner ego ruin your impression in others' eyes. If you work on your mistake, you will excel in your life. Don't lose hope by failing at one time. Keep on trying and trying until to succeed in your task.

# How To Solve Conflicts

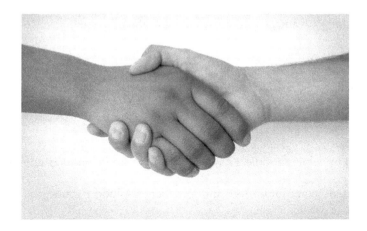

As your toddler increases in independence and begins to exert her will on the world around her, she will inevitably experience conflict. Conflicts may occur with siblings, other children, and adults—including yourself!

Helping your baby learn to manage conflict in safe and healthy ways is vital to his development. Many parents feel that toddlers aren't cognitively developed enough to learn how to solve disputes, instead opting to solve conflicts for their toddlers whenever possible. While there will be times when the safest or appropriate action is for you to take care of a problem from your position as caregiver, there will also be many times when conflicts are an opportunity for you to teach your toddler necessary skills in self-regulation, communication, and social interaction that will provide a solid foundation for more complex situations in the future.

The best way to help toddlers learn how to handle conflict is to allow them to experience it safely, with guidance and support when needed. When done effectively, taking advantage of these teaching moments to help your toddler learn how to get along with others will contribute to her sense of self, improve her ability to self-regulate, increase her social awareness, and help her develop empathy.

The first step in helping toddlers navigate conflict is to be good examples of how to use effective communication and conflict resolution strategies ourselves. Toddlers who see parents yell, argue, become rude or mean, call names, slam doors, etc. are more likely to do those things. Modeling healthy and productive strategies for conflict resolution helps toddlers to develop a healthier and more effective plan themselves.

However, modeling goes beyond simple behavior. It's also a good idea to model thought processes in the moments surrounding the conflict. For example, during a stressful encounter at the bank teller drive-through window, one mother looked in the rearview mirror to see her toddler looking at her with wide eyes. Chagrined, she realized that she'd been more than a little short with the teller.

Before the teller returned to the window, mom pulled out a quick think-aloud strategy: 'Boy, it makes me a little mad that this lady can't help me,' she said. 'But I should be kind so that we can picture out the problem together. I think I'll take a deep breath. Will you help me?' She and her toddler took a deep breath together, and when the teller returned, mom finished the transaction much more calmly. By using a think-aloud strategy, she was able to model positive thought processes that take place in real-world conflict resolution.

As adults, we are often able to resolve conflicts without much help from others. But what about toddlers? How much should we help them solve the conflict?

Toddlers, especially 3-year-olds, are quick to turn to mom to solve conflicts for them. Your response to these requests may range from complete intervention in the case of safety issues, to prompts and guidance as toddlers learn to handle conflict themselves, to be aware but hands-off as you let your little one try to solve the problem on his own.

As long as safety isn't an issue, a good rule of thumb is to let your toddler try to work it out on her own. Doing so will give her the experience needed to internalize successful conflict resolution strategies. However, as you move your toddler towards increased independence in handling conflict, you will still need to stay aware of the situation at hand and be ready to offer guidance in the skills, strategies, and coping mechanisms required to keep safe, respect others and reach her goals.

As you help your toddler learn to deal with conflict, keep the following tips and strategies in mind:

Take a break. Teach your child that sometimes, conflict can be made more accessible by taking a break to calm down. In the beginning, you can simply remove them from conflict situations that have escalated.

Tell them that they 'need a break to calm down' and can come back when they're ready. Before they go back to the situation, make sure they understand why they took a break—to calm down. Later, you can move on to asking them, 'do you need a break?' when emotions start to escalate, encouraging them to regulate their emotions with more independence. Eventually, they may even 'take a break' of their own accord.

Encourage 'I' statements. Teach older toddlers to express the problem from their point of view and to listen to the point of view of others. For example, 'I felt sad when you didn't want to color with me because I just wanted to color too. So I took your crayons to make you mad.' Learning to state and understand the problem will help your toddler understand where conflict has arisen from. It will also help him to become more aware of his reactions. When the problem is clearly stated, you can encourage your toddler to think about choices for dealing with the situation, whether it originated in himself or another.

Make apologies. Encouraging toddlers to apologize after a conflict has been resolved helps them learn to take responsibility for their actions. It can also help them to reset after some intense emotions. When your child is 1, they probably won't be making apologies of their own, although you can model this behavior for them. When they are 2, apologies may consist simply of a single word: 'sorry.' Once your toddler is three, you can usually start directing them towards more meaningful apologies that acknowledge what was done wrong and what will be done better next time.

Problem-solve. If your toddler comes to you asking for help with a conflict, you may want to encourage them to solve the problem themselves. Validate their feelings and ask open-ended questions to get them thinking about what they could do to resolve the conflict. For example, 'Wow, I understand that she took your toy. That sounds frustrating. How could we get it back? How could we find a way to share?' You might suggest compromise strategies or offer guidance, but try to let your toddler choose how to solve the problem. Afterward, praise them for figuring it out themselves.

Step back. Allow your little one to solve her conflicts whenever possible. Taking a step back will allow him to learn from experience. However, that doesn't mean that you aren't aware or active in keeping an eye on the situation. Be ready to offer guidance if needed, but try not to take over unless necessary.

Be safe. Not all conflicts are benign. Watch out for safety issues and intervene immediately if necessary. During the toddler years, you'll especially want to watch out for thrown objects, pushing, hitting, biting, etc. If emotions or behaviors escalate and become unsafe for anyone involved, you may need to remove your child from the interaction. Usually, you can stop things from reaching that point by being aware of the situation and intervening before it gets out of hand.

Acknowledge both sides. If your toddler and a sibling or another child come to you together for help resolving a conflict, don't take sides. Encourage each participant to share their feelings and come up with ideas for solving the problem. Even if one child is clearly in the wrong, make sure that both leave the interaction with their respect intact.

# Consequences From Improper Training Of Your Toddlers

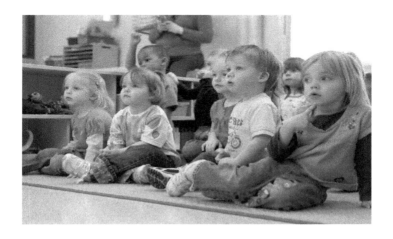

Parents must acknowledge that they are the ultimate reference materials for their children. To this end, the parenting method adopted in the training of the children has long-term and short-term effects on them. According to the 2011 report by the UK's Department of Education, it is understood that the conduct of children who had improper parental guidance is twice as worse as the average child. This was traced to inappropriate parenting done via physical punishment, verbal abuse, coercion, lack of interaction, and inadequate supervision.

1. Greater Vulnerability to Psychological Disorders: In light of a study published in a child development journal, it is understood that children who are directly or indirectly exposed to physical or verbal abuse in their early ages have a higher risk of having psychological disorders. In this study, there was no prevalence when the various psychological disorders are placed in comparison. However, these psychological disorders were all traced to factors in the early stage of children's development. It was found that the relationships with siblings in the family they come from or relationships with their parents had been injured. According to the Child Abuse & Neglect Journal, studies show that children who have been victims of abuse display post-traumatic stress disorder for a substantial period of their lifetime.

2. Defiance to Laws: In light of a research article published in the International Journal of Child, Youth, and Family Studies found that children who suffered parental negligence in their early days were more susceptible to being charged for juvenile delinquency. In this study, researchers were directed to investigate the connection between parental neglect and juvenile delinquency. However, some of the intellectual gaps identified in that study have been filled in other studies. One of these studies is the research published in Behavioral Sciences & the Law Journal. In that study, it was found that mothers who had once been charged with juvenile delinquency commonly

give birth to or nurture children with antisocial attitudes and tendencies to defy laws. According to the study, this was traced to parental abuse and negligence. In such cases, the problems of defiance to laws may be generational.

3. Depression: In the publication titled, "Parenting and Its Effects on Children: On Reading and Misreading Behavior Genetics," Professor Eleanor E. Maccoby of Stanford University explains that one of the causal factors of depression in children is parental adverse reactions toward their children. With these distinctive, credible articles reaching similar conclusions, it is hard to doubt that it is indeed true that factors such as overall support, verbal condemnation, physical punishment, and even depression of the parents are causal to the depression of a child.

4. Failure to Thrive: One of the implications of failure to thrive in toddlers is the retardation of mental growth, physical growth, and malnutrition. According to research submitted to the American Journal of Orthopsychiatry, it was learned that failure to thrive in toddlers is ultimately linked to parental negligence. Children who are victims of "failure to thrive" are found to have lacked good nutrition that is essential for healthy growth. This reduces its average growth rate. A publication in the journal Pediatrics

also traced the failure to thrive syndrome in toddlers to medical child abuse. It is found that parents who impose unnecessary medical treatments on their children make them vulnerable to the syndrome. In cases where your toddlers find it difficult to thrive, you need to check the medical procedures you have been exposing them to and the measure of care you show them.

5. Aggression: According to Rick Nauert's Psych Central article, "Negative Parenting Style Contributes to Child Aggression," the various research conducted by different specialists at the University of Minnesota all had similar conclusions; toddlers who were aggressive and quick to anger all had low interactions with their mothers. The decision was that one of the effects of bad parenting to toddlers is an aggression on the part of the children. The mothers studied treated their children aggressively, were verbally hurtful, and rebellious towards their children. The more negative parenting, the greater the child's aggression to colleagues will be. This created a certain level of hostility between mothers and toddlers. However, more research is now invested in knowing whether or not the relationship of the toddlers' fathers with their mothers influences the bad conduct of the mothers towards their children.

6.  Poor Academic Performance: One of the consequences of parental neglect is the gross reduction in the toddlers' academic performance. This view is credited to a study conducted and published in the Child Abuse and Neglect Journal. The study concludes that when parents have minimal interactions with their children, it impairs the children's' learning ability compared to their peers. The children also lack social relationships. Further research shows that neglect is no less disastrous than physical abuse in terms of the toddlers' academic performance.

According to another study in the journal Demography, children whose parents always relocate or migrate also tend to poor performance in school. The truth is constant relocation is usually a factor that is above the power of the parents. Nonetheless, it may have detrimental consequences on the child's educational growth.

In terms of children's' mathematical performance, research has shown that the parents' mathematical interest can determine whether or not the child will be good at it. According to Melissa E. Libertus, an Associate Professor at the University of Pittsburgh, the connection is said to be either environmental or hereditary. In this light, parents that are easily provoked at their child's academic performance in mathematics should know it might have ecological or genetic causes.

Having seen some of the behavioral, cognitive, and social consequences of improper parenting, it is time you are introduced to a grand principle for training your toddlers.

# Friends & Siblings

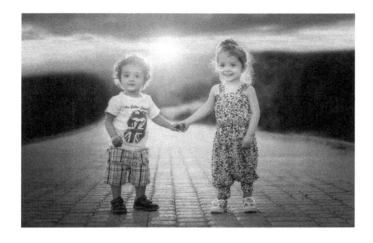

Can small children be friends? They can but in their way. That means you should be prepared to see one bite the other, take the toy without asking. These are things of the age that need to be understood. In the range of 1 to 3 years, the child is still selfish, and the question of the possession of objects is very present. Therefore, it is common for them to take a toy from the other's hand and walk.

The little ones are in the famous oral phase, in which they use the mouth as a means of discovering the world. As long as they do not know how to talk, they end up sometimes hitting for no reason, to get what they want. Of course, if aggressive behavior is too frequent and intense, it requires parental attention. It is unnecessary to deprive the one who was caught up in the other's life but to ensure that it happens in the most secure way possible, supervising and separating in case of aggression.

Not infrequently, a more passive child becomes friends with a bossy one. The experts consulted say that the leaderships of the group begin to dawn with 4 or 5 years. When this happens, others become his followers - and make no mistake about their little age: the leader realizes the strength his opinion has over others.

When the teacher identifies this in school, he should use strategies and jokes to dilute this configuration so that roles are reversed in some situations: followers become leaders, and the leader becomes a follower - this can also be done at home by parents. If conflicts arise from the relationship between a leader and a follower, it is recommended that each child should orally expose the other to how he felt and what he did not like. They should listen and try to resolve the situation with each other.

## Shy Children

More introverted and shy children may have difficulty making friends. In such cases, parents may approach a class in the building's playground, for example, and introduce the child, asking if he can play with them. So, next time, he will already have a reference on how to act. You can also invite classmates to attend your home. That way, they will have what to talk about in the room, plus memories of fun times together.

But if the child is never called to any party and seems to be always isolated, the ideal is to do a job with the school to detect why this happens. You can also enroll your child in extracurricular theatre or sports classes that help decrease inhibition. Just do not press it.

If your child is amiable and makes friends quickly, rest easy. Just be aware of whether your child is not acting that way to get attention and can do a little more work with a classroom concentration. Point it out that there is time for everything.

# Friends – Siblings

Who said siblings could not be good friends? In these cases, one only needs attention if the youngest becomes a" shadow "of the brother and ends up having no personality. Well, then, talk about the importance of having your attitudes.

There are also cases where siblings have no affinity. Parents should be aware of the context in which the lack of friendship happens and their expectations of that relationship. In general, siblings will be friends but often go through situations of jealousy and competition. They may also have different interests, which seems like a lack of friendship, but is related to gender and age. Parents need to look at how they relate to the family (mother, father, and siblings) to identify whether they have a strong or superficial bond because the child perceives and tends to have similar behaviors.

# Leaving

If the parents look back, they'll remember that some of their friends walked away for a while and then returned. You have to stay calm and keep in mind that this is a process of building the child's bond. Another feeling that can arise in such a situation is jealousy. When there is some dependence on friendship, attention is needed. If we identify something negative, that does not benefit both parties. It is necessary to stimulate new friends. The adult should show that the child can discover affinities with several children.

# Outside The Party

This will happen sooner or later, either for financial reasons (it's expensive to invite all the students) or affinity. In these situations, the adult needs to be prepared to face the child and parent's frustration. Parents must accept that it is not the end of the world and explain that some people identify more with each other than others.

The opportunity is ideal for sitting with the child and asking why he thought he was so close to the birthday boy. Sometimes he thinks he's friends with the other, but he's not reciprocated. It is essential to have this understanding that some people give the impression that they are our friends, but they are not.

# Colorful Friendship

From the age of 4, children begin to perceive each other better, start comparisons, and have a more excellent perception of their own body. It is common for situations to arise from one wanting to kiss and embrace the other. Some even talk about dating. This is mostly a reflection of what they see daily in the media, that is, an imitation of behavior. When faced with such issues, parents should teach the child that he can express affection in various ways - with words, drawings, and jokes together - and to say that he should not kiss another person on the mouth.

My son never wants to leave his friend's house. What to do?

Parents should keep in mind that no matter how friendly they may be, there is no way to force children's bonds. The identity that made them be friends does not necessarily happen among their children. And adults should be prepared even to get upset. It would be better to avoid contact between children, especially when there are no others to interact separately. Prefer to date only with adult friends.

# The Friend Is a Terror

You will meet those friends who are a "terror": they make a mess, they mess around the house, they speak profanity ... The desire to criticize the colleague can be enormous. If it is to your child that the message must be given, explain that there are several ways to behave and that the way the other acts do not please you, pointing out how the line has been crossed. The same must be done with swearing. In general, small children do not know what they mean, but if they realize that it causes anxiety in their parents, they can repeat it to manipulate them, just like the tantrum. Therefore, be very calm in explaining that this is not acceptable to say.

# Away From Home

Generally, it is at about four years that the child starts to go to friends' houses and, from 5, can be prepared to sleep outside the home. Knowing the routine and habits of other families is positive, as it broadens the worldview. However, the child will inevitably make comparisons and question aspects such as "in so-and-so's house, I could stay up late. It is an excellent chance to teach your child that each family has its own rules that are not better or worse, just different.

It can happen the opposite; also: your son sleeps there and discovers that he does not identify with the family (schedule, food, fear of a pet). Heed what he has to share and do not force him back. One option to keep the friendship is to take walks with the colleague elsewhere or let your child visit you for short periods.

# My Idol

It is common for children to choose a friend as an idol for a while and want to have the same clothes and toys or repeat their attitudes. Over time, they realize that they do not have to copy the colleague to have their friendship and stop it.

But it is good to be alert when this behavior is exaggerated, asking, for example, why the child wants an object or is doing it. Explain that friendship does not depend on it. If things got worse, ask help from a psychologist. At the other end, the "copied" child can tell his friend, "Be yourself."

# Emotionally Intelligent Parenting

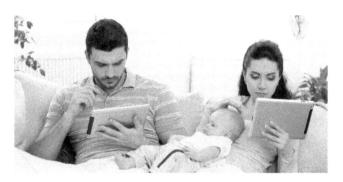

Emotional intelligence is one of the essential skills you need so you can live harmoniously with others. It allows you to get a grip on your impulses and keep a clear head when dealing with conflict. It gives the skills needed to maintain healthy relationships with the people around you. Keeping a tight grip on impulses is crucial when you are raising a child because the most harmful expressions of anger are those that happen instinctively. These include name-calling and spanking an unruly child in the spur of a moment.

## Benefits of Emotional Intelligence

**Impulse control**

Even with a full understanding of your parenting style, you will be hard-pressed to continue acting in a levelheaded way when you are fuming at your child. A person with a high level of emotional control will understand the need to keep their head in charged moments to avoid hurting others. This is what emotional intelligence allows you to become. The higher your level of personal control, the better the power you will have over your impulses. This means that you will still have the presence of mind to take a moment to gather your wits before you start talking or lashing out when you are angry.

## Dealing with crises

Emotional intelligence entails learning how to deal with problems in a sober manner. The ability to do this means that you never have to lose your head when there is a problem because you are confident in your ability to solve it. Feelings of helplessness play a massive part in parental anger, mostly because you are responsible for so much more than your child's needs. After all, the things you do to your child will affect their lives for years to come. The problem-solving technique of thinking about challenges helps to deal with anger because it gives you something to think about and will ultimately give you the solutions you need.

## The most effective problem-solving technique entails;

1. First, seek to understand the exact nature of the problem. Sometimes our fears magnify small issues and make them appear more significant than they are. Define the issue in a statement, then twice more using different words. This allows you to determine what is essential in a situation.

2. Come up with a list of solutions to the problem. Brainstorm as many answers as possible without dismissing any one of them for the time being. Write down these ideas if you are afraid that you might forget them.

3. Go through the different solutions one by one and eliminate those that are non-workable. Narrow down the list of possible solutions until you have the best three.

4. Put the most promising solution to practical use and evaluate how effective it is. If it does not work, tweak a few things and then try out the next solution on your list.

5. Evaluate the whole situation and picture out if you are better off for it. For you to consider a problem solved, the case should improve significantly and visibly.

**Anger and You**

As a parent, you will get a lot of advice from friends and family to raise your child. Some of this advice may work, but most of it will probably not apply to your situation. Even worse, following some well-meaning advice often makes it even harder for you to execute your parenting duties. This is because you make the mistake of thinking that all parents deal with problems the same way. In truth, parenting styles vary and can be as unique as our different personalities. It is just the same way that children have other characters and present problems in unique ways.

# Emotional Intelligence for Your Child

Emotional intelligence is not just a technique that a parent might use to manage their parental anger. It gives anyone who has mastered it the ability to express their emotions transparently and efficiently. It also allows for the mastery of emotional self-control, which means that you can picture out what you ought to say in front of people and those you should hold back. Children usually have none of these skills, and unless you teach your child to express themselves adequately from a young age, they might never master these skills.

Emotional intelligence allows a child to solve problems creatively and put up with others' emotions, especially when these emotions are negative. When you teach your child emotional intelligence, you teach him or her that feelings serve to make us know what we want. This way, a child learns to appreciate his or her feelings and respect other people's emotions. The most important aspect of teaching emotional intelligence is training your child on the practical strategies of dealing with negative emotions.

Parents deal with their children's negative emotions through one of the four methods: dismissing, disapproving, acceptance, and emotional coaching. Dismissive parents put little stock into their child's feelings and try to get rid of them as soon as possible. In a dismissive parent's point of view, a child needs only experience joy. Whenever they display a different emotion, a dismissive parent will use any distraction available to entertain the child back into happiness.

Disapproving parents rarely take the time to appreciate their child's feelings. At the first sign of negative feelings, they do everything possible to quash it by punishing the child. Punishments will often grow harsher as the child's unexpressed emotions grow more robust, and their expression more frequent.

Acceptance is pretty much how permissive parents deal with their children's negative emotions. They accept anything the child does without questioning or seeking to find the cause or possible solution. These parents are also called laissez-faire because they do not teach problem-solving or put any limitation of a child's expressions of negative emotions.

Finally, we have the personal coaching strategy of dealing with your child's emotions. This strategy views every expression of feelings as a teachable moment, and emotional coaching parents will usually take moments of a personal name to connect with their child. By pointing out how doing something can be bad for the child and other people, you empower them to rise above it and learn how to express themselves better.

## Emotional Coaching

Take away from this book and it should be that your child's emotions are essential. This includes the feelings that follow your actions after your child has done something wrong. Children make the most meaningful choices when their emotions are raw.

You must be careful to ensure that these choices are the right ones for your son or daughter.

The five steps for emotional coaching

1. Notice your child's emotions. You must keep observing and reading into your child's actions and words. The best way of coaching your child to manage his or her feelings is to acknowledge them before expressing them. This gives you the time to picture out how best to handle when your child finally expresses the feelings.

2. Take the opportunity to strengthen the connection you have with your child. Find the best possible way of addressing your child's feelings and go with the most fun and pleasurable way of doing it.

3. Validate your child's feelings. No feeling can ever be wrong because all emotions are meant to show us what we need. Try to relate by actually putting yourself in your child's shoes. If you can connect with something from your own life, that might deepen the connection.

4. Clarify what the emotions indicate. As the parent, you are supposed to bring clarity to your child's confusion. It would help if you labeled the feelings your child is going through.

5. Guide your child to solve the problem at hand. The problem-solving step of dealing with negative emotions is crucial for building character. If you handle everything for your child, you risk making them too reliant on

your protection to manage their problems. Focus on teaching the skills

of problem-solving and giving clues rather than providing solutions.

# How To Replace Punishment With Positive Parenting?

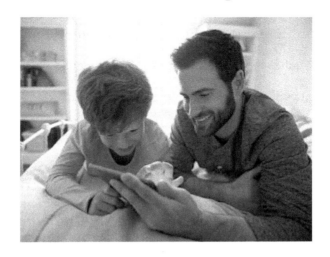

A positive approach to parenthood implies an understanding of the child and his or her behavior, paying attention to how the child feels. What does that mean practically? Seeing what is behind a child, 'child's action means seeing the real cause, understanding it, and offering the child an alternate solution to malicious behavior.

Adults mostly only see the "final product" – the unwanted behavior they want to correct, or a real cause. Suppose they want the child to learn something, and that isn't working. In that case, it is up to adults to explain to the child the consequences of his malicious behavior: natural effects ("You are cold because you do not want to wear a sweater.") and logical consequences ("We are late for the birthday party because you wanted to play even though the clock was ringing and telling us it was time to go.").

Positive parenting requires a calm tone of voice with an agreement and an explanation of what is acceptable and what is not and what will happen if the child does not adhere to the contract. Positive parenting creates a space for learning without guilt, shame, and the fear of punishment.

Children learn by making a series of efforts and mistakes. The whole process of a child's upbringing and learning is a series of attempts and errors until they master some skills. The role of the parents in this process is to provide direction and leadership. You must be a teacher to your children first of all, but a patient one.

Parenting is difficult and requires the patience to repeat the same thing hundreds of times. Being a child is also tricky because it requires strength and persistence to repeat the same thing hundreds of times until it is learned. This process cannot be accelerated, skipped, or eliminated. The least a parent can do is to change their perspective and accept that some things are slow and annoying and have to be repeated many times. Some parents have days when they feel discouraged because they have to repeat the same thing day after day. But that is also a significant part of parenthood.

One of the essential things in your child's learning process is learning how to live in the society in which he or she is growing up and learning the rules to function in that society. Kids have to know when it is proper and better for them to limit their autonomy and self-expression, and they have to know that they can do it. Then, they have to learn how to tolerate frustration and handle frustration and to be consistent despite it.

Without adequate limits in their environment, children feel agitated and unmanaged. Boundaries can be expressed as criticism and cause embarrassment, or they can be uttered in a reliable way - full of respect. Contemplate and speak the same way to your child. Do you respond better to vigorous criticism or respect, regard, and support? It's the same with your child.

If we allow them to, children will try to solve the problems they face in their development and upbringing. Parents often begin to scold or criticize the child, not expecting them to attempt to solve the problem. If the parents were more patient, they would be surprised how much their children can make conclusions and solve the problems they face.

Being heard is therapeutically potent and allows us to think about things clearly and find a solution. The same goes for children. Sometimes it's enough to listen to a child when they talk about their problems because they often come up with solutions that resolve the issues.

Fear and control are useful in the short term. Still, a child can become either completely blocked in his development or can begin to provide resistance to parental pressure through defiance and rebellion. Depending on the type of interaction a child has with their parents, the child forms a picture of himself and a sense of self-reliance in his roles in life. A blocked, non-progressing child has a lesser perception of his value, leading to isolation or it's opposite: aggressive and rebellious behavior.

Children should understand the importance of thoughts and emotions, not just behavior because it will enable them to function better in relationships with other people and deal better with problems. That is why adequate control of their emotions is an important skill, and one of parenting's most essential goals.

The words of parents and their assessments of a child are a mirror for that child. Children will see what their parents exhibit. That then becomes their picture of themselves, and they live with that. That is why it is essential to be specific and accurate with criticism. Criticism should be expressed with body language, which expresses regret rather than disapproval toward the child. The child will internalize a parental look full of condemnation and criticism, and we want to love and accept our children. This strong support for them will be the seed and the core of their happy life and success.

However, you should 't shouldn't give your child unlimited freedom; you do need to discipline them, of course. But how? Disciplinary measures respond to the child and his abilities and support the child in developing self-discipline. Discipline aims to target children, recognizing individual values, and building positive relationships positively. Positive discipline empowers children's faith in themselves and their ability to behave appropriately.

Discipline is training and orientation that helps children develop limits, self-control, efficiency, self-sufficiency, and positive social behavior. Discipline is often misunderstood as punishment, especially by those who apply strict punishment to make changes to children's behavior. Discipline not tantamount as punishment.

Instead of punishment, children need to be provided with support in the development of self-discipline. Positive discipline shows adults as pictures with authority that children allow developing strategies to control their behavior according to their age. Parents should take e a positive approach to discipline, developing positive alternatives to punishment.

Education is based on establishing and building relationships with your child, and the basis of each connection is acceptance, respect, and established boundaries. Setting the boundaries during your child's education is equally important as understanding, love, and support. In this way, children learn to be responsible for what is happening to them, and they are helped to learn self-regulation of their feelings and behaviors, gain self-confidence, and feel the confidence and trust of their parents.

Children know what is right and what is not. This is the knowledge that they adopt, and their parents are the ones who assist most in this. It's a formidable job, and children need the support of adults during this process. Parents need to learn how to stay patient and calm and help their child to learn in the best way possible.

# Tips and Solutions for Peaceful and Positive Parenting

1. Speak in a calm voice - Rather than shout, talk with your child. This will help you to understand how kids need to feel a bit more of your patience. The way you react always influences the way the child behaves. Use positive parenting because it is vital for a healthy relationship between you and your child.

2. Give yourself a break - Patience is time-consuming. Sometimes it's hard to understand why your child behaves in a certain way and what you can do to help them. Patience is difficult when you have no time, and your child wants something from you. Patience is the power of understanding your child.

3. Try to understand your child - Understanding is the foundation of positive parenting and influences communication and respect. It is effortless to lose patience with a child you do not understand. Your toddler will always be a little nervous, tearful, angry, or just loud and not listening. However, you're a parent with unconditional love. If you ever try to talk to your child based on this unconditional love, you will surely understand him better and become more patient.

4. Let your child be independent - If you want to practice patience, put it to work in situations where you want your child to take on tasks for himself. Stop and allow the child to finish things. This is how the child will enjoy independence, and you, at the same time, will learn to be more patient.

5. Find the fastest way to calm yourself down - This is one of the most important things to learn about patience. Ways that can help you—for example, deep breathing. You can also count to 10, bake a cake, or something like that. You know what you can do to bring about quick relaxation.

# The Power OF Empathy

Being an empathetic parent is the best gift a parent can give to their child. Your empathy for your child will let them understand that you actually 'get them.' Just like adults need someone to show confidence in them and acknowledge their feelings, so do young kids, especially toddlers. We need an understanding shoulder to lean on and cope with our time of distress. That shoulder will only be supported when the person understands where we are coming from and the reason for our present situation.

Toddlers are no different. They need us, parents, to be those understanding shoulders for them. We can become such strong support for them only by showing empathy. It is essential for kids that we understand them and their needs. For toddlers, their emotional needs and their feelings are of paramount importance. For us, a crying, whining, screaming, thrashing child might be just that, a child behaving undesirably. More so when according to us, they are doing so for no real reason and 'nothing.' But for them, it is hugely important. How many times have we encountered parents who defend their ignorance of their child's needs by saying it was 'nothing'? For us, it indeed might be nothing, but to them, it is as essential as the world.

Being empathetic toward your child gives you the space to see the world through their eyes. It makes space for your feelings without any judgment. Empathy is the great affirmation that toddlers need that tells them, "I understand how you are feeling. It's alright. Your feelings matter to me."

Empathy lets your child feel connected to you. It gives them a sense of belonging and security. They will be more at ease, knowing you are someone who understands them. This will bring more confidence in your relationship with your child. Children who have empathetic parents are more comfortable to "manage" and workaround. They live with the knowledge that they have support to fall back on bad days. If the parent is always critical and lacks empathy, the child will retreat within themselves. Such parents may be unable to foster a relationship based on trust and confidence with their kids. Such children will build resentment toward parents as time goes by. Empathy gives them the validation their feelings need.

Their mistakes are welcoming the very first step to validation. You are not accepting their behavior, instead of embracing that they are humans and will make mistakes just like you do. We are taught that mistakes are wrong from our early childhood, and the ones committing errors are wrong. We are taught that making an error is akin to failure. Children are innocent. They aren't bad, and they are pure. But when we are not welcoming of their mistakes, we are saying the exact opposite to them. When you are accusatory in your approach, kids resort to hiding and covering up their mistakes because they fear you. Hiding mistakes can never be a good idea, as one lie would need a hundred more to hide it. This is not a good trait to encourage in your child. When you hide wrongdoing, you can neither rectify it nor learn from it to avoid it in the future. Instead, be welcoming of their mistakes, guiding them gently to correct them with empathy. This is what validation gives them; a chance to get back up from their failures, learn from them and try not to repeat them.

# Validation Versus Acceptance

Many parents confuse validating their child's behavior with accepting their behavior as correct. These aren't the same. The proof is to affirm the feelings of your child as something worth taking note of. You give their emotions the respect they deserve without brushing them off as inconsequential and meaningless. One of the biggest criticisms of empathy theory is that it encourages the child to feel confident about their mistakes and urges them to continue their bad behavior. This also isn't true.

Validation is not equal to condoning bad behavior. You are validating the way your child feels but not the way your child behaves. While you are empathetic toward your child by telling them how you understand their feelings and why they are angry or upset, you also firmly establish how you do not support or condone their bad behavior. See the following as an example.

A three-year-old is upset that her older brother has finished her orange juice. They both get into an argument, and she throws the empty juice carton at her brother, who ducks, and the open box lands on the side table, holding crockery, breaking a glass quarter plate and smashing it to pieces on the floor. Their quarrel and argument have resulted in a broken plate and the danger of strewn glass pieces all over the kitchen floor. Any caregiver would be angry. She was in the right by being upset, but was the ensuing argument and throwing things appropriately? How must the parent react? How would you react?

What the child needs here is for us to understand that firstly she is simply three years old. Just two years older from being a no-idea-what's-happening infant. Only one year older from being able to talk. That is still a very young age for us to be taking them to the task. So what do we do? What that child needs are a hug and a rub on the back that tells them you understand. If it is a sensitive child, they would be crying even before you look at them. A more authoritarian child is bound to melt into your arms and call when you give that hug. Why is this so? Because at this tender age, kids are too innocent of fostering any real hate or negativity. Their guilt will bring those tears on. They are too overwhelmed by the loss of their juice and then the loss of their own emotions. You would only be hurting them more by scolding or yelling at them.

Once they have calmed down, the crying has subsided, and they can look at you without being uncomfortable; now is the time to tell them it was wrong gently. By this time, they know that already. But you have to lay down the rules when your child is calm and in a receptive enough state to listen and acknowledge what you are saying.

"I know you were upset. You were angry; your brother drank your juice. But, dearest, what just happened wasn't fine. You mustn't throw things at each other. We talk about and solve our problems. We do not throw things at each other. This could have seriously hurt someone."

This much is enough to let the message sink in. But this message will only get in their minds when you have held them and rubbed their backs, giving them that much-needed hug. That simple, empathetic gesture broke the barrier between the parent and the child. It is what made the child more accepting of their follies and the given advice. Of course, you mustn't forget the older brother or his part in this whole scenario, but for now, our concentration was the vulnerable little girl of three.

Validation is like saying I get how you are feeling. I'm afraid I have to disagree with what you have done, but I understand why you have done it. You can and must set behavioral limits while being empathetic at the same time.

# Strategies on How to Empathize With Your Toddler

If you are looking to be empathetic to your child's feelings, there are a few things to keep in mind to convey the right message of understanding effectively.

- Bring yourself to their level. Either bend down or kneel so that you both are at the same level.

- Look your child in the eye and truly listen to them. Put away any phones or electronics, or any other chore that you might be doing, to give them your undivided attention.

- Reflect and repeat what they say. It is always a good thing to repeat what they tell you back to them. Doing this accomplishes two things. It means them you have understood what they are saying and opens for them a chance to correct you if you have misunderstood them.

- Describe how they look and give them words to help them tell you how they feel. For example, you may say, "You are pounding the table with your fists; you look angry!"

- Ask them appropriate questions, so you know you understand them correctly and validate their feelings and not the feelings you have chosen for them. For example, you might say something like, "You look sad, are you sad?" And then you let them agree or disagree.

- While being empathetic, do not criticize, judge, or try to solve their problems. Doing this would only defeat the purpose of being compassionate in the first place.
- Do not tell them, "You are feeling sad, so this is what you need…"
- Do not tell them, "Stop crying. If you go on crying, everyone will think you are a cry baby."
- Do not tell them, "You are always upset at the table during dinner."

Validating your child's feelings is just as important as teaching them manners and ethics. For toddler years, this is even more important as at this tender age, they are unaware of the complex emotions a human being is capable of feeling, and all that they undergo is bound to be overwhelming for an innocent mind. This age needs the most amount of validation and empathy to help the child learn the range of their own emotions and handle them.

## Have a Meaningful Talk

Sometimes all you need is to sit and talk. Make it a point to have at least one meaningful conversation with your child every day. What you could do is have such a discussion at bedtime with your child. Before or after storytime, you could sit with your child and talk about your day. Then ask them about theirs and listen. It is remarkable how much a child is willing to share when you are ready to listen. Ensure that you end your conversation on a happy note that leaves your child smiling. Be it a joke, a funny story, a funny incident from your day at the office, or anything else, let the last memory of you be a happy one for your child as they drift off to sleep.

Having such sharing sessions is a step toward empathy. It will help you strengthen your relationship with your child and enrich the trust factor between you both. This is a valuable asset to have in your relationship as a parent as your child grows. With time, as your child grows and starts school, this same session will come in handy. Your child will be more forthcoming and trusting of you to share their day with you every day. This ease of conversation is what any parent desires, and you can have it too through a little empathy.

# Teaching Your Child To Problem Solve And Be More Independent

There were so many times I have wanted to fix all my sons' problems. But I knew that I couldn't because I would only be holding them back instead of helping them. I want them to depend on me, come to me, and ask me anything. This is one of the biggest reasons I, like you, want to jump up and do absolutely everything I can for my children. As you do, I also know how this can keep them from going out in the world with confidence and learning from their mistakes. After all, making mistakes is one of the most significant ways we learn, grow, solve problems, and become more independent.

I understand when you struggle to take a step back and watch your child try to picture a new toy. I know how hard this is because it pains us emotionally to see our children struggle. However, I also know the thrill you and your child feel when they can overcome an obstacle. We often have tears in our eyes as we tell our child, "Good job! I am so proud of you!" I know I teared up when I've watched my children succeed. It's what we dream about as parents, even the little successes.

# Tips on Teaching Your Children How to Problem-Solve

To do our best for our children, we often focus on the various information we receive from other parents. Therefore, I will share tips with you about how you can help your child learn problem-solving skills at any age.

**Give Your Child an Obstacle**

Giving your child a roadblock sounds like the opposite of what you want to do. However, think of it this way – if you can place an obstacle in front of your child, you can strategically. This means you can think about your child's problem-solving skills and make sure there is a solution for them to picture out. This will help them build their confidence when it comes to solving problems and allow you to see them thrive.

**Don't Hover Over Your Child**

I know we all want to do this. It's hard to see our babies grow up – actually, we always consider them our baby. But if you want the help, your child succeeds, you will know when you need to back away and let them take care of the situation themselves. For instance, your child comes home from school and tells you that another child pushed them. You look at your child and, while you want to go to your child's defense, you take a deep breath and ask them what they did. Your child responds, "I told them that isn't nice and not to do that again, or I will tell."

At this point, you still might want to hover over your child and go to school the next day to inform the teacher what happened, but you know it's more important not to at this time. Instead, you focus on praising your child because you are proud of how they handled themselves. This tells your child that you care about what happens to them, but they can also take care of themselves. It also gives them the confidence to know how to handle people who are mean to them compassionately and politely.

Another way we can find ourselves hovering over our children is by not giving them enough space. This not only includes independent playtime, but the freedom to make mistakes, picture out what happened, and learn from them. Toddlers will need a little guidance when it comes to figuring out their mistakes and learning how to change their behavior or actions, so the error doesn't pop up again. Helping your child in this way is not hovering. You start to approach when you stop your child from making a mistake.

## Make Problem-Solving a Positive Experience

Everyone runs into problems daily. We all have issues we need to solve. We might not always see them as problems, but they are there. Take time to reflect on your days and notice what problems occur in your life. Then, think of your toddler's days and their struggles. Picture out ways that you can turn everyone's problem-solving experience into more fun and favorable situation. For instance, if your child comes to you with a problem, look at them and say, "I see your problem.

Why don't we think of a couple of solutions together to help solve this problem?" With your toddlers, you can also make this into a game. For example, if they like Sherlock Holmes, they can play Sherlock, and you can be Watson trying to solve a problem.

**Do-It-Yourself Projects**

There are tons of do-it-yourself type projects for people of all ages. While your child can help you with home improvement projects at times, there are also smaller projects that you can work on with your child. You don't need to make sure that you do everything correctly or don't ask for help. Your child is going to learn more about solving their problems by watching you solve yours. Therefore, if they see you ask for help, they will understand that everyone asks for help. If your child sees you make a mistake, they will know that they can make a mistake, and everything will be okay.

Along with these types of projects, you can also look into puzzles. By the age of four, your child has probably put together tons of puzzles, which is a way that helps them problem solve. Continue to buy your child puzzles, but make sure that they are age-appropriate.

# Problem Solving By Ages

## One-Year-Old Problem-Solving Skills

While one-year-olds who are closer to two might start helping you put puzzles together or shapes in the correct spot, most of their skills are going to happen through observation. Have you ever stopped to think about how often a one-year-old will sit and watch other people? This is because the primary way they learn and start to develop their skills is through observing, listening, and taking in what is going on around them. At the same time, their mind is busy processing all the information they are taking in.

One of the best ways to help your one-year-old develop problem-solving skills is by showing them how to do something. For example, your child received new stackable blocks from your sibling. At first, they look at the blocks and seem puzzled. They might pick up a block and observe it more closely. At that moment, they don't understand that the blocks are meant to be stacked on top of each other. Therefore, you will take the time to show your child how the blocks work. Once you do this, hand the blocks over to your child and watch them mimic your actions. It's always an adventure to see how your young child catches on to what you have shown them so quickly!

**Problem-Solving Activities**

- Play a variety of accessible games for one-year-old children that will build their problem-solving skills, such as blocks and puzzles

- Playing peek-a-boo.

- Use objects to play hide-and-seek. You want your child to find the item. They are learning that just because they can't see an object doesn't mean it doesn't exist.

**Two-Year-Old Problem-Solving Skills**

At two-years-old, the memory comes onto the stage and gives your child a whole new way to learn how to problem-solve. This is a great age to start to bring easy puzzles and games, which will help build your child's problem-solving skills. Just like a one-year-old, the most significant way two-year-olds are going to learn is through observing. The only difference is; they are going to remember what they saw for a longer time.

Your child wants to color. They have asked you to help them get their crayons, but you are in the middle of preparing supper, which means that your hands are greasy and full of food you don't wish to get on the drawer where the crayons stay. You tell your toddler, "Go ahead and open the drawer, and you can do it." At first, they look at you, at the drawer, and look at you again. They have never opened the drawer before, so they are a bit anxious about getting it open. You assure them that they will be able to open the drawer just fine. "Open the drawer as I do," you tell your child. They then walk to the drawer as you start to wash your hands. You know that they have only been able to shake and bang the drawer to open it. They have never opened it before, so you are preparing to help your child. However, your child surprises you, and perhaps themselves, as they pull the handle and open the drawer without too much of struggle. "Look at what you did, baby!" You exclaim as you clap with your child's excitement.

At two-years-old, your child will use their memory to think about ways to solve a problem. They will start to come up with solutions in their mind and then see if this solution works. This is often why two-year-old children will stare at the problem before they try anything. It's not because they are becoming frustrated or thinking about giving up. They are trying to picture out how the toy works. The best step you can take is to observe your child. Notice their facial expressions as they are thinking and get an understanding of their thought process. You will also want to keep them so you can ask them if they would like to help if they become frustrated.

### Problem-Solving Activities:

- Teach your child how to play "Simon Says."
- Use words like "over," "under," and "above," as this will help your child picture out what these words mean. They are great words to use when your child is looking for a toy that might be under the table.

- Gets toys and puzzles that let your child sort pieces through shapes and colors.

**Three-Year-Old Problem-Solving Skills**

Three-year-old children will often show a look of focus, yet they will become frustrated. They will use memory to solve problems but are more prone to trial and error than a two-year-old child. This is because three-year-old children will try things their way more than through observation or with help from their parents. This is also one reason why many people say that threes are worse than twos. It's because your three-year-old toddler will try a variety of new and exciting problem-solving skills while you are in another room. You won't have a clue what they are getting themselves into until you walk into the place for the surprise.

# CONCLUSION

*Thank you for reading all this book!*

Adults ought to build conditions that fulfill fundamental development needs for identity, competence, freedom, and compassion to raise responsible and productive children. They identify these "four paths" as the Circle of Courage. There is clear proof that the needs of the Circle of Bravery are based on fundamental ideas, and perhaps even on the human DNA:

1. Relating: The child's need for human attachment is nurtured in confidence partnerships so that the kid can believe in "I am cherished."

2. Mastery: Training to deal with the environment boosts the child's inborn appetite for information, and the kid can say, "I will excel."

3. Independence: Increased responsibility nurtures the child's free will so the child can believe "I am in charge of my life."

4. Kindness: The essence of the infant is nurtured by empathy for all, such that the infant will say, "I have a life meaning."

In Western society decades, parents sought to raise decent children by teaching them to be compliant. Adults that claim compliance will set minimum standards, determined by the level of loyalty. Both children require people surrounding them who are compassionate, supportive, committed, and trustworthy if they are to thrive entirely. We have to become the immediate family of ancestors and parents that once encircled every boy.

*You have already taken a step towards your improvement.*
**Best wishes!**

# Toddler Sleep Training

## The No-Cry Sleep Solution for Toddlers and Preschoolers

Written By

## Jennifer Siegel

# Table of Contents

# INTRODUCTION

*Thank you for purchasing this book!*

There is no doubt that raising a child is hard. When they are babies, they may require much of your time for feeding and cuddles. But, once they become toddlers, they will reach a whole new level. This is more than just gaining the ability to move around; a toddler is naturally curious and has no real knowledge of the dangers they will face, so you need to guide them and lead by example.

As parents, we often think that social skills are something our kids will naturally pick up the more they mature. This isn't true. Ask yourself this, have you never met a man or woman you wished had some more manners? Maybe they cut you off in a grocery store line or overtook your car on the highway. Perhaps they lost their temper in front of you or had poor control over their emotions. Maybe they lacked basic table manners and created an orchestra of sounds while eating with a fork and spoon, or perhaps irked you with the way they flossed their teeth later with a tooth-picking stick. Gross! I know, right? It is in these moments that we realize the importance of good social skills.

The desire for independence: To become a responsible adult, your child must move slowly from the passenger seat to the driver's seat and learn to drive the tortuous paths of life.

For children, everything is black or white; for example, for a child, the concept of justice is simple: 'Mama broke a cookie and gave half to me, half to my brother.' In this case, justice comes down to a mathematical formula. Abstract thinking helps your child draw their or own conclusions about complex issues. But this has a downside: their findings may be contrary to yours.

*Enjoy your reading!*

# Sleep Training A – Z

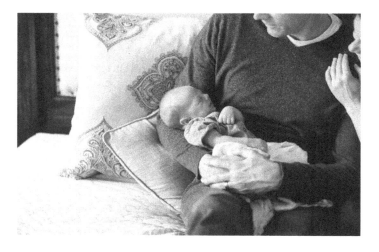

When your baby comes home from the hospital, the chances are that you will have the baby sleeping in the same room as you. It's practical, and it's the best way to ensure that the baby is safe. It's also an excellent way to have access to the baby for feeding. If you can place the cot near the bed where you can reach out and get the baby for feeding sessions, this is the best way to do it because it minimizes interrupted sleep. When the baby has been fed and is ready to sleep again, he can be placed back in the crib to sleep. Be aware of his need to be winded and also the need to rock the cradle until the baby has gone back to sleep.

The majority of this book is about toddlers, and they are quite a different story. You may have the toddler in your room for a while until you have prepared a place for them, but if this is the case, make sure that you involve the child in the preparation of his/her room so that they look forward to a time when they have their own space, rather than worrying about it. When a toddler is placed into bed, he/she needs to be tucked in. Then, you need to turn down the lights and read a story to the child. If the child gets out of the supine position, put him/her back into that position and continue with the information.

The routine that you use should be the same as is used every night, and if there are times when you are not going to be there to do that, it's a good idea to explain to a babysitter so that the babysitter can do what the child is accustomed to. The whole bedroom routine and training consist of the following elements:

- Getting ready for bed and putting toys away
- Bathing and putting on pajamas
- Cleaning the teeth and brushing the hair
- Going to the toilet/ or at least changing diapers
- Getting the room ready for the night and closing the drapes

The toddler needs to know what is going on and should trust it. If you change the routine too many times, the toddler can get disorientated and very irritable. Particularly boys find a change in pattern demanding for their minds to cope with. Thus when you are training a toddler, from day one of the way surrounding their independent sleeping should take on the same format. Encourage the child to enjoy the room that is theirs. The one thing to remember is that the psychological factor does come into it. You cannot place a child in the bed and then leave and close the door. The child needs to be settled. Place the child into the ground, lying down, and start your storytelling. It's a good idea if both parents can take part, but if this is not possible, the child should at least be allowed to say goodnight to both parents.

After the story, the child should be encouraged to look after the teddy or the toy that the child has chosen as his friend. If you work on the basis that the bear is smaller than the child and needs all the love the little one can give him, the child will respond well and be happy to be tucked in with the toy. This is an age when a child doesn't understand much about relationships except for what he learns during his playtime. You can use the teddy to give examples of good behavior and make the bear into his trusted friend. That way, when bedtime comes, the toddler does not feel all alone in the world when the door is closed for the night.

It's a good idea to have the light ready for the night before the storytelling so that the child's eyes get accustomed to the room's dimmed light. You can have a baby monitor in the room, but don't make a big deal. Just check that it is switched on and that it is monitoring the baby. If you have already set the angle, you don't need to play around with it. When the story is finished, and the bear is tucked in with the child, a kiss goodnight seals the deal for some kiddies, while others may cry for attention if this is the first time they have been left their own. There is a way to get the child used to the cot, and you can do that during the daytime when it's nap time. Close the drapes and make the light dimmer but carry on doing housework around the child's room and adjoining area, so that he gets used to the fact that you are not far away. What this does is help the child to trust the cot environment.

If the child does cry and you feel that it is warranted to check on him/her, then open the door slightly so that you don't have to make a lot of noise going into the room. It's a mistake to turn the light on or make a lot of noise as toddlers have oodles of energy, and all you are doing if you change the room's ambiance is wake up that energy. Talk to the child in a whisper and tuck the child in again. Listen to what he has to say. Don't be too quick to leave the room. You can sit by the cot for a while so that the child knows that you are there. Little by little, as the sleep gets more in-depth, you will be able to move out of the room, and the chances are that the child will sleep for the rest of the night.

One thing that you should be aware of is that children do tend to wake when daylight happens. It's not that they have a built-in clock yet, but once they have had a decent night's sleep, their energy levels are higher again, and you may find that difficult at first, but you will get used to the rhythm of their day, little by little. You should establish with a child from baby age the difference between night and day and open the drapes to greet the day. It takes a while for a child to understand the sleep cycles that they need to go through. Their body clocks have not yet adjusted to life, and by making a clear distinction between night and day, you are teaching them how life works and allowing them to find their rhythm to life.

# Sleep Training Tips - Cheeky Chops

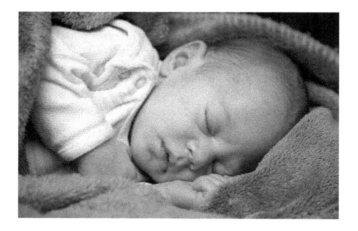

Before electricity, people would rise and fall with the world's natural light source, which fit in with our standard biological clock - in those days, numerous people got the required sleep. Today in our quick paced 24-hour society, our capacity to keep up adequate quality sleep is enduring - ask yourself where rest on your rundown of needs is?

This is consistent with for kids and infants - with such a large number of classes and exercises to take an interest in - numerous children, toddlers, and Mum's are overbooked. A portion of these classes conflicts with a tyke's familiar plunge in sharpness, so normal snoozes become increasingly difficult to set up. More sleep is required in early stages than some other age gathering, and the absence of sound sleep for infants and kids is hindering physical and emotional well-being; it ought not to be disparaged.

The most significant test for most guardians is how to get this quality sleep for their kids; if propensities are now instilled, the possibility of influencing changes to can appear to be overwhelming with such vast numbers of current schools of thought, consolidate this with your very own sleep hardship and the entire idea becomes amazingly overpowering.

Most importantly, you have to choose what you and your family see a healthy sleep routine to incorporate - what are you OK with and not happy with. Try not to feel forced to make changes due to outside sources. Make the right decision for your family.

It is conceivable to make changes with the relevant information and direction - however, don't expect awesome outcomes quickly - be reasonable. For youngsters who, as of now, have affiliations or have a multi-layered issue, sleep preparation is a learning procedure. It is done in stages to influence the progress to go smoothly for everybody. It requires investment, ingenuity, and, above all, consistency. Envision endeavoring to find out how to play an amusement someone steadily continued changing the standards - you could never find out how to play the diversion - isn't that so?

**Here is a rundown of inquiries and tips to consider before making changes to your family's sleep.**

Do you have a day by day schedule? Youngsters flourish with consistency. If you never knew it would occur or when you would next eat or sleep - how might you feel?

In what capacity can your baby or child fall asleep? If your newborn child uses support (shaking, Mum or Dad's chest, chest, bottle, etc.) when your baby is in light rest, they will have brief edification and consistently need comparative conditions to come back to rest. These results in no rest for all social occasions included. In what manner may you feel if you slept in your bed agreeable and alright with your duvet and pad and woke up on the front nursery?

Where does your infant sleep? Pick one spot where your infant can sleep - ideally a lodging - this is where they should take most all things considered and all evening sleep. OK, feel all around rested if your sleep area shifted - vehicle - carriage - lounge chair - sling - swing?

What time does your youngster head to sleep? Missing your kid's regular break is fundamental when you need a simple change. An overtired tyke regularly acts wired and once twisted up, is exceptionally difficult to settle. Do you feel languid after supper and afterward get a second wind later at night?

Does your kid snooze regularly? Do whatever it takes not to care about the criticalness of daytime sleep barely. If your youngster is always missing rests, their capacity to adapt in their surroundings diminishes, and afterward they virtually emergency. How might you change when you are exhausted after a long clamoring day and are preparing dinner, with the phone ringing, the TV on, organizing tomorrow, and endeavoring to watch the children? I am sure that you have a craving for shouting, much the same as a tyke does.

Making changes to your infant or youngster's sleep ought to be done when no other significant life changes occur with the goal that you can think and give devotion. It's not reasonable for your infant or tyke to continue changing strategies or techniques - this will prompt perplexity.

At the point when is it a Good Time to Move Toddlers to a Bed?

The word bed initially the territory where an individual sleeps. Initially, a foundation was very little more than an opening in the ground. The primary sort of infant beds was supported; they were little and well-fitting for a newborn child. Child beds have a rich history. They were more than likely one of the essential household items brought into a home when the child's updates were coming.

Amid the 1800s, when houses increased, the bassinet came to be as they could bolster a developing kid's necessities. They were commonly custom made and after that go down from tyke to kid. Child beds were additionally passed on to more up-to-date ages of children since they were worked from the solid wood of the region in all probability.

When is a decent time to move your infant from its support or den?

When you see that your infant exceeds its den, you should move the child to the giant bed. Numerous children take to sleeping in a large bed in a flash instead of sleeping in their support. A lodging is made for newborn children and little kids. There is no hard-quick principle for a particular time to move a child out of favor and into a den.

By and large, supports become unreasonably little for an infant in its third month. To energize peaceful sleep, you may wish to move the infant into a lodging right now. If your infant exceeds its support right now is an ideal opportunity to move the person in question into the bunk.

Infants develop and, in the end, begin moving about; if your infant is moving the bassinet, it can become dangerous to the tyke. Since little kids don't comprehend gravity's consequences, they can't shield themselves from falling if the bassinet turns over.

Keep in mind not to put any pads of stuffed toys into the bunk with your kid since they can present dangers of surrendering to abrupt newborn child passing disorder of SIDS. When you leave pillows and toys in a bed with a young child, they can cover death. You ought to be cautious in your choice of an infant bed, with the goal that you are not jeopardizing your youngster while endeavoring to think about it appropriately.

You can roll out the improvement from a support to a den much smoother for your infant via preparing it to appreciate the distinctive bed. You do this by enabling the tyke to entertain themselves amid the day while watching you from the securely of their lodging.

If you search for incredible blessing thoughts, you may wish to consider one of the many infant blessing crates. You can discover them on the web. Some you will probably pick and pick the kinds of endowments you need to be incorporated into the blessing bins you purchase for an infant. You can select a customized infant blessing bushel today. Regardless of whether you are picking a blessing crate for a young lady infant or a kid infant, you are sure to please the youngster's mother just as picked only the correct presents for the infant in need!

# Characteristics Of A Bad Application Of The Discipline Or Errors.

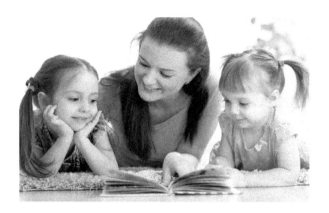

Perhaps we will ask ourselves why to address the issue of mistakes or the wrong application of the discipline, because, in my opinion, it is essential since as it is said, "From mistakes you learn," or on many occasions we do not we realize them and repeat them regularly, this does not mean that we are bad parents or bad educators, what it tells us is that we can improve, it is also appropriate to mention that throughout this writing not only the errors will be mentioned but also aspects of how we can achieve effective discipline.

Parents and educators can adopt defined styles of education, and that in many cases are not the best, which can have consequences in the child, since many times

21

methods are used that are at the extremes and do not reach a midpoint, there are a series of ways that do not give significant results, which are:

- **Rigid Methods:**

Through this, the images of authority parents or teachers have all the power and the rules, that is, they are too strict, consequences are not administered, but punishments, the needs of the child or opinions are not taken into account in this model adults are right. There is no discussion since the child is only trained to follow instructions, obey. Perhaps the child behaves "well," can be given security, stability, and predictability, which can be considered as advantages; however, What is achieved when they grow up is that they are toddler without initiative, the little capacity to make decisions, little creativity Also that responsibility is not encouraged, this toddler may become rebellious, have low self-esteem or be dependent on the opinions of other people.

- **Permissive methods:**

This method is opposite to rigid, the expression is given way, the creativity develops, the feelings, opinions, ideas of the child are taken into account, and the opportunity is given to make the decisions about whether or not they do homework, if they want to help in the housework or not, etc., That is, few or no rules are established, they also do not administer consequences because it is believed that the child will learn from experience, however in this method it is not taken keep in mind that the child cannot self-regulate their behaviors and make long-term decisions, this can generate anxiety, insecurity, reduced capacity to meet their needs and do not recognize the importance of things, often these toddlers grow up and fail to adapt to social norms and are frustrated by the lack of tools to face life, since with this type of education no skills are created, and toddler lack structure to achieve goals.

- **Combination of methods:**

Many parents want to find the midpoint and seek to move from rigid discipline to permissive. Vice versa, when stiffness does not work, they pass to permissiveness and do so indiscriminately, which causes insecurity, inconsistencies, extreme contradictions in the child and the child does not He manages to understand how he should act or not act, because, at times, we want the child to respect our authority. At other times we allow him to do what he wants.

# Methods Used By Our Parents.

Sometimes parents, as they do not know how to handle their toddlers, decide to take the pattern that their parents used with them; however, as we were part of that process, we did not like as toddlers as we did not apply it. If we wanted it, we used it. Still, many times, what worked out is what was not pleasant for us. However, it is essential to realize that generations or times are different. Each child is other and has its own particular needs, so the toddler seems more to the age that has to live than their parents.

**Copy some methods used by another person.**

Sometimes we do not know how to react and use the method used by another person, and it has worked. It may be possible that if you have given the results that the person expected, however many or most of the time, it does not work because they are different circumstances, and the child has its characteristics.

**Errors That Parents Commit Frequently**

As we can see, there are various ways or methods of educating that is inappropriate for the toddler, in addition to many of our behaviors as educators or parents do not cause a proper development of the child or on the contrary, they cause damage, so I will mention some mistakes that we can make discipline toddler, in which we can work to improve as parents or educators.

Reacting based on impulses and emotions can be shared in educators, only act without thinking. You can hit or harm a toddler physically and emotionally, since it is only about resolving the conflict that you have at the moment, without reflecting and realizing what happens, in what circumstances is happening, and how I can face it so that it is not recurrent.

The strategies we use with toddlers are sometimes excellent. However, there is no time for them to give results, and it is continually changing to get what we are looking for quickly; however, the solutions are not always immediate; sufficient time must be provided and perseverance to work; For example, a child does not like to do homework, and we make him see that it is his responsibility and he has to fulfill it. If he does not achieve it, he will not perform any of his favorite activities, for example: playing, watching television, going to recess, etc. This is usually a good strategy, but it doesn't work because we expect the child to learn and do his homework for the first time, and he doesn't need us to be consistent and constant.

Many times it is not known how to react to the behaviors or attitudes of the toddler, which causes them to be undecided before them, and this is usually a mistake since toddler perceive it, this affects their feelings of safety and well-being, being authorities Indecisive can allow the child to be inconsistent and dominant, which provides the child with the chance to do what he wants, without respecting rules and regulations.

There are many behaviors or behaviors that we want to change in toddlers. However, we do not analyze the causes or nature of the actions that we want to change; this is why our change strategies do not work, it is necessary to investigate why this behavior arises, and from there, we will find a way to solve it, for example, if a child tantrum when going to the store why not you buy candy, what we do is buy the candy to avoid tantrum or crying. However, we do not realize that the outburst will occur every time the child wants something since this gets things and on the contrary, what we must do is teach the child that characteristics can be obtained without tantrums and sometimes it is not possible to buy the candy or get what he wants.

For convenience, laziness, lack of self-discipline, or simply because they learned it from their parents, they follow a teaching pattern. They do not want to change, which is usually a grave mistake because, as mentioned before, the toddler is different from others; in addition to the natural development of the child, it leads us to the need to change these behavior patterns, which we find challenging. We prefer to continue as until now because despite not being the most convenient for him, it is what that I know and has helped me achieve what I have so far. Still, it is essential to realize that the important thing is to adapt to their needs and characteristics.

Some educators, mainly the parents think that while the child is small, "you have to save him work, because he will have to fight later", that is, activities or tasks are done for the toddler, or on the contrary he is not allowed to help us in the work because the child is a bit awkward and does not perform the activities as we would like and sometimes it takes us longer than if we do it for ourselves, this is a very big mistake since the child is not allowed to learn to persevere and be responsible, what is achieved with these attitudes is that they are lazy, spend time wanting to rest and killing time on things that will not be useful, or on the other hand it is demanded of more, the toddler must carry out activities according to their age and their real capacities, since if it is not so the child will always be frustrated by not being able to perform the entrusted activities, which will generate him insecurity and anguish, it is, therefore, essential to know the characteristics of toddler and to know at least in a general way the child development.

We may have a misconception of love for the toddler; many times, we do not let them do anything for fear of what may happen to them. We do not allow them to be bothered, and we do not let them take risks that are sometimes necessary for their development; we would like to keep the child in a glass bubble, as it is commonly said "we do not want the air to give it," we consent too much. We may mistakenly believe that what we are doing is the best. However, overprotection, instead of showing the child how much we love him, creates an insecure, shy, indecisive creature, accustomed to others acting and deciding instead.

Introducing fears is to disarm and limit the child, it is essential to realize that fear disorganizes and weakens the mind, inhibits, creates shyness and also damages the psyche, many times we as educators are afraid of something and transmit them to toddler, this It is we teach him to fear something that he did not worry, this fear we can make it increase or decrease if we are altered we cause the child to improve his fear, and if on the contrary we are calm and give him security this fear will diminish little by little, on the other hand, fear is also instilled in the child to gain control over it, many times the child is told: "if you misbehave, the devil takes you," old," which does not lead the child to learn something productive, on the contrary, it is harmed, and this is often done by not hitting or scolding them. We believe it is the best solution, but it is necessary to reconsider and find other ways to maintain control of the kids.

# Listening Types

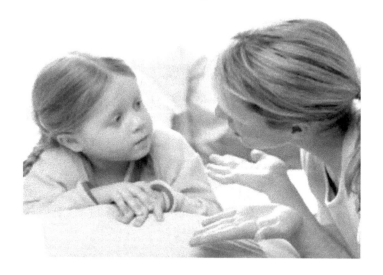

Now that you have learned a bit about how the listening process works, you can begin to discover that there are many different ways to listen. This is something that you already understand.

There are many different ways to listen, and you will probably display a general tendency towards some ways over others. What is important is that you realize that each type of listening has its merits within a specific context. To become a good listener, you must be receptive to the context and listen properly. This is part of the active listening process, a position which shall be named here, dynamic listening.

Active listening occurs when you actively adapt the listening you engage with depending upon the context, as you see fit. This depends on the environment, as well as the individual needs of the speaker. You would not, for example, be displaying the best listening behavior if you turned up for a lecture listening only to the emotions of the speaker.

Applying the most appropriate type of listening is an important skill.

# Undesirable Types Of Listening, Or Non-Listening

Before you overthink about listening types, you must develop a sense for your non-listening behaviors and undesirable listening types. Everyone has these habits, but to become more of an active listener, you have to become more aware of negative patterns that may be holding you back.

Pseudo listening- The clue is in the name! If you are displaying pseudo listening traits, then you may be giving all of the feedback that implies that you are listening, such as smiling and nodding in agreement now and again, but your attention is on your thoughts. There can be many reasons for this, whether it be a lack of interest in the conversation or a pre-occupation with your ideas or on tasks that you must accomplish for the day.

To eliminate pseudo listening, admit your lack of attention as soon as you notice it rather than masking it with fake signals. Just say "sorry, I wasn't listening," or

"I don't know where my head was then, please can you repeat that bit," or something of the like.

Selective Listening- Selective listening is related to our perceptual barriers, which can screen out what is being said. When our bias is so extreme that we only hear what we already agree with, or what we already know to be true for ourselves, then we are selective listening. This listening flaw can prevent us from learning lessons and from understanding incoming perspectives.

Example: You are against the consumption of meat. A friend starts to tell you about why they enjoy eating meat, and why they don't think they could be vegetarian. Instead of listening to their reasons and trying to understand their perspective, you blank out what is being said. You only really listen to one bit if the conversation, the bit where they say, "I do wish I could be vegetarian." This bit suites your bias, but represents only a fraction of their message, which was intended mostly to express their passion for cooking with pork.

Defensive Listening- This type of listening behavior always assumes the worst in a conversation! When you are listening defensively, you are presuming that someone is saying, or is going to say, or is implying something terrible about you, when in reality, this is not the case.

Listening defensively often creates a conversation with little understanding and lots of conflicts.

Example:

"I enjoy eating pork, that's the problem."

"You mean you like to murder animals."

"I just find it difficult to eat lettuce all the time like you."

"I'm not a rabbit. We eat very well."

"You don't eat that well, and you have no protein in your diet."

Combative Listening- Combative listening is the harmful listening habit that most people will be able to relate to in a big way. When you listen in this competitive manner, you are only listening for the gaps in the conversation, so that you can take the lead in speaking again. As soon as the speaker even starts to talk, you are busy formulating a response and looking for an opportunity to say your bit.

Example:

"I was looking at this great blender the other day...."

"I have a blender, and it does me wonders."

"Yes, so I was thinking about buying it..."

"Mine was only £50, and I bought it straight away."

"See, I was unsure whether to buy it, so I..."

"You should have bought it. If it were anything like the one I have, you would have loved it."

# Understand The Message Of The Speaker

It is much better to listen to the full message before responding and to base your responses on what the speaker is trying to communicate, not on what you are desperate to say. Active listening is a matter of focus on understanding what the speaker is saying and listening to their feelings where it is appropriate. Combative listening, like the other negative listening behaviors mentioned here, doesn't care much for the speaker. When you listen in these ways, you are effectively only concerned with your response, your own beliefs, and opinions, or your insecurities.

# Are You Listening In The Right Way?

Take note of any fixations or listening preferences you have, and try to work out whether there may be times when you have used a specific type of listening in the wrong context.

**Informational-**

Informational listening is used when your purpose is to pick out relevant information, to learn something new, or to help you to accomplish a goal. Examples of this include listening to a lecture, watching a "how-to" video or documentary, or in a work setting where you might have to follow specific instructions. This sort of listening should primarily be dominant when you are being instructed, or when you are taking in new information that you want to learn.

When someone has something to teach you, be willing to learn, and be ready to listen.

Examples of contexts where it is appropriate to listen informationally:

listening to a talk or lecture

learning something at work

learning how to play guitar off a friend

taking instructions on a task from your parents

learning how to wash your clothes (children and husbands alike)

taking a yoga class

watching a how-to video, and so on

**Critical-**

Critical listening occurs when the purpose is to evaluate or criticize or to make a judgment about what is being said. It is used for problem-solving and decision making. Critical thinking is analytical; it helps you make informed choices and formulate opinions based on what you hear. If you find yourself weighing up the strengths and weaknesses of what is being said to you, you are engaged in critical listening.

Critical listening is essential in a wide range of contexts, and socially it is useful in most conversations in which a specific topic is being conveyed. It is particularly favored by those who like to debate or learn by challenging others' views. If you have loved ones who enjoy this sort of conversation, then critical listening is the basis. By listening to the other person's argument or belief, you can draw on your analysis of it and respond with your ideas.

Example:

"I think that you are suggesting that the shopping center is genuinely good for the community, but I tend to disagree. I think it is bad for local business."

"You say it is bad for local business, but quite a few shops still thrive."

"Yes, they thrive for now, but how long will they last?"

**Appreciative-**

Appreciative listening is when you find yourself listening to something or someone only for enjoyment. The most straightforward example of respectful listening is when you listen to music or poetry. You enjoy the sounds as they move over you.

A typical response to appreciative listening is to show approval for the story, music, or poem, by clapping, laughing, or verbalizing pleasure. You could proceed to tell another level in a conversation, one that the other person can sit back and appreciate.

**Empathetic-**

Empathetic listening occurs when the purpose is to understand the feelings and emotions of the speaker. When you listen in this way, you virtually try to share the speaker's thoughts and want to come to grips with their perspective, even if you don't necessarily agree with it. In this case, you have to listen to the content and the feeling of the message. In the case of loved ones, this often involves a certain amount of reading (or listening as it were) between the lines.

This type of listening is highly desirable and is something that you should try to cultivate for yourself. It is incredibly beneficial for your relationships with those you feel deeply for to learn to listen in an empathetic way.

Examples of contexts when empathetic listening may be appropriate: when your children are talking about their day at school, when they are expressing their feelings about something, when your spouse is upset when your friend needs someone to talk to, and most conversations that involve anything more than informational listening, or debate for debate's sake. A certain amount of empathy always goes a long way in most contexts.

**Therapeutic-**

Therapeutic listening goes beyond trying to understand the feelings of the speaker, though this is a pre-requisite. In therapeutic listening, you use your empathetic connection to help the speaker change, understand, or develop somehow. It requires the same receptivity to emotions and feelings as in compassionate listening.

Examples of contexts when therapeutic listening might be essential: where negative emotions are involved, when a loved one needs some emotional help or advice, when someone needs to be encouraged to open up, when a loved one is sad, grieving, or has lost someone, or experienced hard times.

**Dynamic Listening**

Active listening is the idea that you should try to engage in listening to that matches the communication context. So, if the speaker aims to inform you on how to fix your computer, you desire to hear in an informational way, picking out relevant instructions. Suppose the speaker is seeking to start up an intelligent discussion about politics or society. In that case, you listen critically, analyze their trail of thought, and think about how their opinions are related to your own. If the speaker wants to express their emotions, be it sadness, anger, or ecstasy. You aim to listen in an empathetic or therapeutic way, allowing them to vent their feelings and provide support on an emotional level.

# The Most Effective Method To Move An Out Of Control Toddler – Parenting Oppositional And Defiant Toddlers

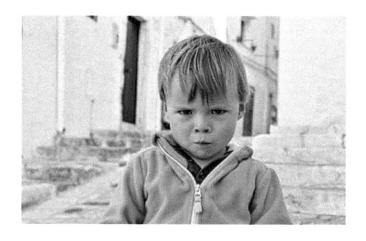

Knowing out how to move a wild little child is nobodies most loved past time. This can be a troublesome yet extraordinary little circumstance. Child-rearing oppositional and resistant toddlers are dependably a test. Anyway, when it comes time to move them, it very well may be incredibly upsetting. Children can be forceful and fiercely crazy at the same time when they become overpowered.

This is entirely ordinary; however, to the extent, formative benchmarks are concerned. Not all children who display these symptoms have Oppositional Defiant Disorder. Children at this stage are unpracticed with how to deal with their feelings.

The first standard is never given in or gives them what they need. If you have ever been stuck in that terrible open fit of rage tossing baby circumstance before, at that point, you realize you need to move them. Or, on the other hand, instead, expel them from any place it is you are.

This isn't, in every case, accessible. Shockingly it is fundamental much of the time, however.

It's in every case best to think about the quantity of the people around you and comprehend not every person will be annoyed by it. Still, instead, it's preferable to be protected over grieved and evacuate your child. A standout amongst the ideal approaches to move your wild little child is via completing them face supporting their middle. You put one arm through between their legs and coming to up to get your other arm behind them and head.

It is a lot simpler to encounter when you carry another person alongside you. They can offer some help and assistance. Counteractive action is dependably the best power, yet here and there when they are experiencing these stages; they can be entirely capricious; thus, it's challenging to stay away from. Youthful children, particularly toddlers between 3-5, have an exceptionally troublesome time managing dissatisfactions and controlling their more grounded feelings.

It tends to disappoint when you consider it incorrectly. So, endeavor to comprehend that the vast majority are not taking a gander at you in a revolting judgmental way. Nobody will scrutinize your child-rearing abilities either. A natural 90% of people completely comprehend what you are experiencing and are not, in any case, worried in the scarcest. If anything, they are most likely relating with compassion and upbeat in the learning they are not the only ones since they agree with their children.

They can be entirely extreme with the punching and kicking, so it is continuously encouraged to hurry once you see the signs. If they are now kicking and jumping, proceed and rapidly overpower them by taking a few to get back some composure of their arms. Support them securely and afterward move quickly for the entryway. At whatever point you see this written in books or magazines, the expression is quite often, "Tenderly however immovably." I like it, however. It works.

Child-rearing oppositional and insubordinate toddlers aren't typically entertaining, mainly when they leave control in broad daylight. At that point, it moves toward becoming time to move the shouting, kicking the baby. It even sounds hazardous — we as a whole need to do what we should to help them through this stage. Tolerance is significant and dependably recollects that the more you give in, the more they will rehash this cycle.

# Bad Words

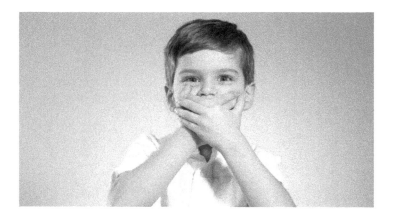

They pop out of your child's mouth at what seems like the worst moments. He or she appears to be announcing to the world that you are a terrible parent and that you have exposed him or her to terrible things. They are going to let everyone know that they heard those words, even if they have no idea what they mean.

It can be a complete shock the first time that your child drops a potty mouth bomb, especially when it is in front of friends or family. We spend so many years trying to help them build their vocabularies, understand what words mean, and watch every word we say in front of them when all of a sudden, this filthy word pours out of your baby's mouth as if he or she has heard it since birth.

The first thing that you need to understand is that no, toddlers have no idea what these words mean; they only understand that somewhere they heard someone use one, and it was used in an emotionally charged situation.

Toddlers will pick up on these words very quickly. Often, it only takes them hearing it one time for it to stick in their little heads and pop out of their mouths when you least expect it to.

There is no way, no matter how hard you try or how protective a parent, you are that you can protect them from learning these words. It does not matter that you do not use them in your home, chances are that the child is exposed to someone that does use these words or they are exposed to the child of someone that does use these words. They can hear them on television; remember, they may not always be utterly asleep as you are watching your favorite television shows in the evening. They can listen to them slip out of your mouth as you are cut off in traffic, or they can learn them from the kids in daycare. No matter what, these words are always there, and just because they pop out of your toddler's mouth, it does not mean you are a terrible parent.

Your child is merely mimicking what he or she heard someone else say, and they are trying to find out what happens when they say it. One huge mistake that I see parents do is that they burst out laughing, whether it be from embarrassment or whether they think that it is funny when their child blurts out a bad word. This is a huge mistake because it is teaching the child that you believe what they did is funny; it is encouraging them to do it in the future and not teaching them that they should not talk like this.

One thing that taught me very early on not to use these types of words, especially in front of my children, was that studies showed those who used curse words were of lower intelligence than those that did not. I never wanted to be the type of person that came across as lacking intelligence, so I did my best to ensure these words did not come out of my mouth.

I am sure that you do not want yourself nor your child to give the appearance of lacking intelligence, so when these words come out of the child's mouth, it is essential that you do not laugh or make jokes about it but instead, show the child that it is a serious matter.

Curse words are not the only lousy language that comes out of a toddler's mouth. Toddlers often begin using potty language, well, when they start potty training.

We have to remember that toddlers can be rude, they can be mean, and, even though they do not mean to be, it is simply not acceptable behavior. We have to nip it in the bud before it gets worse.

When you begin potty training, you must teach the child that words such as poop need to remain in the bathroom. You do not want to suffer the embarrassment when your child announces to the cashier at the grocery store that she smells like poop simply because he or she knows that word will get a reaction out of you.

That is one of the main reasons that children use potty language; they know that this type of language is going to get some reaction out of you, and they are using it as a means of controlling the way that you react. This also happens when a toddler begins using swear words and sees that they can get a huge reaction out of you.

The best way to stop this type of behavior is to start at home. When you hear the child say a potty word, you need to let the child know that this is not how we talk, that the specific name is either not allowed or that it is used to define a particular bodily function and nothing more. Do not react as if the world is going to end because your child said a word that they may not understand. This will only encourage them to continue speaking this way in the future. Instead, remain calm and explain to the child that they are not allowed to talk about that way and that it is not polite.

You have to keep a poker face on when your child says a swear word or a potty word. When a child learns that they can make an adult laugh, angry or upset, they are going to continue to display the behavior simply because they saw that it got a reaction out of those around him or her.

Even if the child invents a new word, and you think it is just adorable or funny such as 'poopy face snot breath,' do not laugh. Do not smile, and do not encourage that type of talk. Let the child know that it is not acceptable and that they should not speak that way. Use a low tone of voice, showing the child that you are disappointed in the way that they were saying. The child is going to understand quickly that you disapprove, and even if he or she was trying to be funny, chances are it is not going to happen again anytime soon.

It is also essential for the child to know words that will allow him or her to express themselves without using curse words or potty language. For example, if you notice that your child is using potty words to express his or her anger, teach the child how to say, "I'm mad."

Never take the time to explain what swear words mean to a toddler. The toddler does not need to know. Instead, if the toddler is stuck on a swear word, and no matter what you do, will not give up the name, you are going to have to get a bit stricter and start doling out discipline when the term is used.

Since the child does not quite understand what empathy is yet, it is going to be hard for them to know how a simple word can upset someone. However, you need to explain this to them, especially if the story that they are saying could be construed as racist or derogatory. Again, you do not have to tell the child what the word means, but let the child know that the story causes hurt feelings and is not pleasant to say.

Above all, it is essential that you watch what is coming out of your mouth. How do you ever expect your child to understand that it is not okay to say bad words when all they hear coming out of your mouth are bad words?

Take the time to expand your vocabulary, find a different way to vent your anger, whether it be through exercise or even writing in a journal. Once you stop saying these words, you will be amazed at how simple-minded other people sound to you when they are spewing them out of their mouths.

There is no more significant step that you can take, which will ensure that your children are not using curse words like this one. I encourage everyone out there who is reading this book and dealing with or worried about dealing with a child using swear words to start paying attention to what is coming out of your mouth.

It is also essential that you pay attention to the language that other adults use around your children. Of course, there are going to be those rude, obnoxious people in the store or out in public that feel everyone around them needs to hear their filthy mouth. If this is you, STOP. No one wants to listen to these words come out of your mouth!

When this happens, as a parent, it is difficult for us not to say anything. However, instead of getting into an argument with someone about the way that they are talking in a public area, just let your child know in a quiet voice that this is not how we speak and that those words should not have been saying.

What about when it is someone that your child spends a lot of time with? This can get a little tricky, but one thing that we make sure that all of our guests know is that swearing is not allowed in our homes. It is not just a rule that the children live by, but it is a rule that everyone who walks in our door must follow as long as they are in our home.

This leads to the question: What if we are in someone else's home or on an outing with a friend? Most people would be respectful if you simply tell them that you would appreciate it if they watched what they said when they were around you and your child.

Everyone that knows me knows that they will not hear a curse word come out of my mouth; for that reason, they are meticulous when they speak in my presence because they know that I find these words offensive. This also means that they are careful about what they say when they are around my children.

When your child sees this, the child will understand that the person is respectful of you, and that is the last thing I want to talk about; you need to teach your child to be compliant. Not just when it comes to the words that come out of their mouth but in all of their daily life.

The way that this is done is to be the example that you want your children to follow. Lead them by example, teaching them how to treat people and not to gossip about people behind their backs, how to be kind, and share with those that need our help.

# Handling Toddler Rough Spots

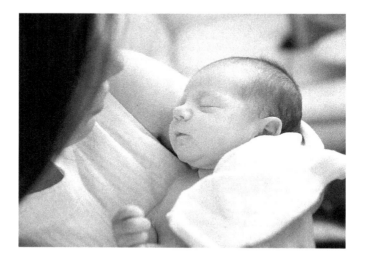

Every toddler has rough moments. One minute they are playing happily—the next, they scream and throw toys across the room. As parents, we must navigate these rough spots with caution. It is not only for the sake of our sanity but also for the toddler. It's important to remember that many children have unwanted habits as they grow—from mood swings and a hostile demeanor to stubbornness and even biting—toddlers challenge their parents.

# Know Your Little One's Triggers

If you have ever been running low on fumes, either tired from not getting enough sleep or moody because you have missed a meal, you might understand where your toddler is coming from when you have a rough day. The best way to handle rough toddler spots is to avoid them whenever you can. Make sure that your child has time to eat and drink before you leave the house. Don't drag them out to go shopping during the time that they usually nap, even if you are running short on time. Be aware of the things that upset your child and try to avoid them when possible. Keep yourself armed with drinks and snacks if your little one gets hungry when you are outside of the house.

# Handling "Bad" Toddler Behaviors

Even with a preventative defense, toddlers will have those days where they do not want to listen. They may be focused on achieving their own goals or put in a situation where they do not know how to handle their emotions. For example, hitting or biting another child should not be encouraged—but it is a natural reaction when your child feels 'anger' after another child takes their toy. By handling these 'bad' behaviors well, you guide your child to better choices. Even when they are undesirable, it's important to remember to shame the behavior and not your child. They are not bad for biting; the action of biting is terrible.

# Dealing With Throwing

Throwing can be a problem if your toddler is throwing things at other kids or continually making a mess. Often, throwing happens for one of two reasons. The first possibility is that your child has discovered the magical effects of gravity—everything that he or she throws falls instead of up. Balls bounce, and spaghetti splats nicely on the floor. It is also possible that your toddler is throwing because of aggression. It would help if you approached discipline differently, depending on your child's motives.

# Dealing With Interrupting

Toddlers believe they are the center of the universe. It does not matter what time of day it is or what you are in the middle of doing, but they want their parents to realize this, too. Toddlers take it so far that they constantly interrupt their parents, doing things to distract their parents from what they are doing, and bring their attention back. However, keep in mind that toddlers may not be interrupted on purpose—they want you to be interested in them. It can be frustrating, but you should avoid using discipline or yelling to set them straight—then you are just giving them the attention they wanted.

# Dealing With Running Away

Toddlers run away for one reason—they want to exercise their independence, and after a year or longer of not being able to walk on their own, their legs can now carry them across long distances. Unfortunately, running away is a severe problem. In the moments when a toddler slips away, they could become lost in a crowd or run across a crowded parking lot and get hurt. A toddler could be yards away within the seconds that a parent is unloading their sibling or pulling a stroller out of the trunk.

This is a behavior that cannot go unmonitored. As toddlers age, they can run farther—but with just as much danger as they faced when they were younger. The best defense is preventative here. If you take off running and screaming after your child every time they run away, they may start to think that it is a fun game you are playing.

# Dealing With Mood Swings And A Bad Temper

Some mornings, you know that it will be 'one of those days' with your toddler. They scream because their juice was in the wrong cup, they don't want to watch their favorite show, and they are not in the mood to do anything you want them to. This can be a frustrating situation for parents, but it is essential to look at their bad mood from a place of perspective. Have you ever been running low on fumes, going through emotional upset, or even just hungry and taken it out on someone else? Maybe you snapped at a coworker who asked you for a favor or was more frustrated than usual when your toddler dumped their crayons all over the floor and refused to pick them up. If adults are not entitled to foul moods, then why shouldn't a toddler be? Toddlers go through emotional turmoil many days as they grow into their emotions, learn what they feel like, and handle them.

## Dealing With A Headstrong Toddler

Headstrong, stubborn toddlers are hard to deal with. They do not have a sense of time or time, and they want what they want when they want it. When their parent fails to deliver, it can lead to fits, tantrums, screaming, or a simple refusal of doing what their parents want. It can be disastrous when your toddler is headstrong. Instead of dissolving in a pile of tears like your child or resorting to yelling, there are a few strategies you can use to guide them to the right choice.

## Dealing With Screaming

Toddlers may scream for several reasons. Sometimes, toddlers cry because they are frustrated or not getting their way, and they are trying to make someone understand that they are upset. Others, toddlers are loud simply because they can be—learning what to do with their voice can make them exuberant and loud. Excitement can also cause screaming in toddlers.

# Dealing With Whining

Whining happens when a toddler feels powerless. They raise their pitch in higher and higher tones, hoping that their parent will pay attention to them. This is not usually done intentionally—they feel they are not being heard, and they don't know how to communicate that you aren't listening. Their frustration at this situation comes out as whining.

# Dealing With Tantrums

Temper tantrums, screaming, and whining are generally forms of attention-seeking behavior. While your little one might throw a temper tantrum when they are angry, they are just as likely to throw a tantrum when they are not getting their way. Once they have your attention, they are often sure they will contact you to cave in to their wishes. Unfortunately, when a toddler continues with the tantrums, many parents give in. This only teaches the toddler that if they raise enough of a fuss, they can have whatever they want.

# Dealing With Aggressive Behaviors

Aggressive behaviors are more common than parents think. They are often shocked by aggressive behaviors, especially when their child is hurting someone else's. They may not realize the reason their child is hurting a pet or another person. The reality is that there may not be a reason at all. Toddlers are still learning autonomy, which is how their own body interacts with the world around them. They may not understand that they are causing pain by being aggressive. Even so, aggressive behaviors can damage social opportunities and be a problem if they are allowed to continue.

# Aggression And Social Development

Parents often think their toddlers have poor social skills, especially between 1 and 2 years of age. The reality is that toddlers often lack social skills this early in their life, regardless of whether they have siblings or are around other kids a lot. Of course, being around older kids helps a little—but only if they are patient with them.

While most parents associate scratching, biting, hair pulling, and hitting with behavior that children should NOT do, it is 'normal' at that age. Many kids do not enjoy the company with others, and their limited social skills can cause them to react in an undesirable way. The best thing to do? Remove your little one from the situation, especially if they are younger than two. They may not have the impulse control or the social skills to share with another child or take turns. They also have not yet developed sufficient problem-solving skills to develop a solution when they are upset.

# Dealing With Lying

Toddlers who lie often do not realize their wrongdoing. Even though allowing your child to lie can cause problems in the future, it is essential to remember that toddlers are young. Their minds are not always developed enough that they can distinguish between a truth and a lie. They may 'lie' for any number of reasons, including:

• They don't want to get in trouble- When presented with a tense situation, they may be reading into your body language. This means that they will deny it when you ask them if they were eating the cookie—simply because they can tell that eating the cookie was 'bad.' The reality may be that your toddler lacked the impulse control not to eat the cookie once he stumbled across it. They are not intentionally lying about eating the cookie—they are scared of the repercussions for this 'bad' thing they have done.

• They believe they can do no wrong- As parents often let things slide when a toddler is younger, especially since they are still learning the rules and expectations of the world around them. While this is good for development, toddlers also think of themselves as incapable of doing wrong. They may lie about accidents or mistakes they make, simply because they see themselves as inherently good.

• Forgetfulness- Parents often forget that toddlers have limited short-term memory. While you might have only been out of the room for ten minutes while your toddler scribbled on the wall, they may have scratched and forgotten. This means when you confront them about it, they may not remember. Even when they do remember, it is not uncommon for toddlers to hear your tone of voice and fall prey to wishful thinking—they wish they hadn't made all those marks on the wall so much that they convince themselves they didn't do it.

- Active imagination- Sometimes, children are not lying—they do have a pet frog that sleeps under their bed and imaginary fish that go with them wherever they go. Remember that toddlers repeat what they believe is the truth. It does not matter whether it is true or not.

# Mistaken Goals At Home

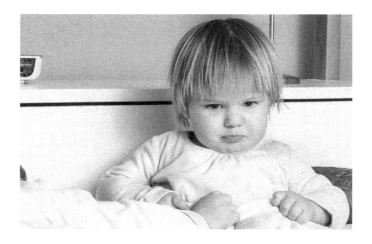

A kid who is misbehaving is trying to communicate with us. Because of his needs, whether it's physical or emotional, are not fulfilling. The mistaken goal is a term referred to as understanding why students are misbehaving. When a kid feels that you are not fulfilling his needs, he will turn to the "mistaken goals."

These goals are called mistaken. Yes, mistake because these are a try by the kid to get his desired thing. And there are four primary wrong goals that you will see in your kid. And the only reason behind this is to fulfill his need.

These mistaken goals are power, attention, inadequacy, and revenge.

# Power:

Power is a fundamental mistaken goal. A kid wants to be a boss and wants some space. If you are giving him too many instructions, that can trigger this goal. In this case, firstly, help him in understanding the situation. Secondly, encourage him to do what he is trying to do in your supervision.

# Attention:

Is your kid misbehaving to get attention? Observe this when he is misbehaving when you are around or not. Is he misbehaving with everyone or only with you? Analyze the situation. Think about it. Are you spending enough time with him or not? For a kid to measure your love towards him is the time. The much quality time you will spend with him means you love him.

If you feel your kid is trying you to notice, he pays attention. Spend extra time with him. With this, you will see a positive change in his behavior.

# Inadequacy:

When your kid is tired of something or hopeless, he moves towards the inadequacy goal. In this goal, a kid gives up and wants to be alone. He intends to disconnect himself from others. At that point, as a parent, your kid needs you the most. Tell him you are there for him and he can't give up.

# Revenge:

When something hurts the kid in its reaction, a revenge goal emerges. Kids are sensitive; anything can badly hurt them. It can be your harsh comment or anything. When he gets hurt, he started to misbehave others. And the reason for this is to take revenge and to show his anger.

# Strategies To Redirect Behavior:

As a parent, yelling or punishing is not the solution to control the kid's behavior as these situations can escalate his action. There are three strategies or steps to redirect a kid's behavior.

# Check Your Behavior And Emotion:

As a parent, you need to check your action and emotional status. Have you yelled at kids when you were stressed or tired? Have you negated him frequently? It is essential to keep a check on yourself before reacting. If you are in stress and not available for him emotionally child's behavior will escalate. Therefore, it is essential to redirect his action to make yourself emotionally available to him.

# Listen And Understand What Your Kid Is Trying To Say:

Kids cannot clearly describe their feelings. You need to understand what he is trying to communicate. As a parent, it is a challenge for you to understand him. But unfortunately, in some cases, parents get frustrated. That frustration hurts the kid's behavior. Thus, understand your kid's behavior goal and deal with it with affection and care.

## Understand The Need Of Your Kid:

To understand the kid's feeling and needs is the most critical task. Don't fulfill all their unnecessary needs. But at least listen to them. Show them you care for them. In a shopping center, the reason for their crying can be to get something. But one thing you are ignoring as you didn't listen to him. It can be another reason. Like he can be tired or hungry. Or maybe he is sleepy.

Therefore, to redirect the kid's behavior, full-fill some needs. Besides that, understand his unmet need and his feelings. Talk to him about that thing. Tell him the right and wrong about that thing. And yes, if you are making a promise to him, fulfill it. Never break your contract and give him that thing as a gift on the promised day. With this, he will trust you and your promises.

# Mistaken Goals In The Preschool

These goals are associated with specific feelings. For example, a kid with loneliness might misbehave to gain attention. But the way of seeking tension can be unacceptable. Similarly, the reason behind an angry kid is to show he is powerful.

Unfortunately, in preschool teachers, teachers also adopt these mistaken goals as they think that they are powerful and right. And the kid is wrong, and they can control him. But on the other side, the kid also feels the same. He thinks he is right, and he is strong enough to deal with the teacher.

This tussle between students and teachers creates a mess and an unhealthy environment. You will not accept that you are wrong when you will be angry. Likewise, students also get frustrated and feel anxiety and shame.

# Mistaken Goals And Feelings:

The primary wrong goals are connected with emotions. Like the false goal, "attention" is associated with loneliness or isolation. "Revenge, Power, and Control, who's right and who's wrong," is connected with anger. Besides this, "Avoidance of failure" is associated with shame and anxiety. Similarly, Withdrawal-Avoidance-Relief is related to depression, guilt, shame, and anxiety.

A teacher needs to recognize the mistaken goals in students. And not only in students but also in themselves. Because only then can they deal with the students positively and healthily.

# <u>Behavior Is A Very Thing:</u>

Teachers should understand that action is not a problem. It is very thing. Deal it as a symptom, not as a severe problem. In other words, it is a reaction to a dysfunctional amount of emotions or thoughts. The only thing a student needs in that situation is your help. A teacher needs to keep the student's history in front of him. And after proper observation and understanding, she needs to handle it gently.

• "You Can't Come to My Birthday Party: Social Skills for Preschoolers:

Social skills are the skills we use to communicate and interact with others. Daily we met with the people and shared with them. Similarly, kids also meet with their peers and communicate with them. But it is also a fact that nowadays, even kids bully their peers. Based on their likes and dislikes, they talk to their class fellows.

With coming to school, kids start to make new friends. Some kids love to make friends. While on the other side, some kids never want to talk to someone. They never want to talk to them and never share their things with them. It is essential to teach the kids social behavior through social skills in school because this training or learning will stay with him for the rest of his life.

# Vital Social Skills For Preschoolers:

There are some critical and significant social skills. Parents need to reinforce them at home and teachers at school. Because of the reinforcement of these social skills being substantial, you cannot teach these skills to kids. But yes, you can reinforce these skills by showing it to them through your actions.

**Sharing:**

Sharing is an important skill. See whether your kid is sharing his toys or snacks willingly with his friends. There are various studies available on the sharing behavior of the kids. And these studies showed that from one to 3 years, kids mostly share their things. But when they have stuff in quantity.

While from the age of 3-6, kids are a bit selfish and are possessive about their stuff. Especially when it comes to a thing that costs to themselves; for instance, if he has only one candy, and you asked him to share that candy, he will be reluctant. Sharing is essential as it helps the kids to make new friends.

Develop the skills of sharing in your kid without using force. Give him incentives and appreciate him when he shares something with others. Make it a habit to reinforce him to share whenever there is an opportunity.

## Caring:

For kids caring is an essential social skill. From an early age, they need to learn compassion for their siblings and others. Teach the kids that when someone is in pain, don't laugh as it is unacceptable. They need to help them, whether it's a human being or an animal.

## Communication:

The communication at the early stage of children is not proper. Most of the children hesitate to communicate. Even they avoid doing eye-contact with others while talking. They need to have communication skills. As in their future, it will help him in all aspects of life. He must know how to communicate with full confidence. He must use non-verbal communication appropriately.

In communication skills, tell your child the difference between rude and polite communication. Teach them essential words at the age of 4 to 5. The words like thank you, sorry, and please. Make yourself a model for your kid. As at this stage, kids try to copy others rather than listening to you.

## Listening:

Your kid's behavior, learning, positive discipline, everything depends on listening. Without listening skills, a kid cannot learn anything. Besides that, he cannot excel in his life. A kid is born with listening skills, but you need to polish and enhance it.

To improve his listening skills, you can play various games involving listening skills and, for instance, whispering a word or telephone without wrong signals. With these simple games, you will see improvement in your kid's listening skills.

**Group activities:**

Teach the kids to engage in group activities. It will help him to work as a group member in his later age. As these are kids, so design such games that can be played in a group. With this activity, they will learn other things, too, like patience as they need to wait for their turn. They will listen to them carefully and will respect others.

# From Crib To Toddler Bed

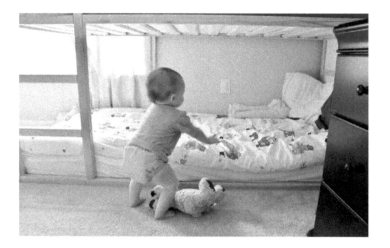

Cribs are recalled due to safety defects and hazards from time to time, so check with the manufacturer before making your purchase. When conducting your inspection, watch for the two common problems. First, the slats shouldn't be more than two ⅜ inches apart so children can't get their head caught between them. Second, make sure older models weren't painted with lead-based paint.

## Sleepy Climbers

Cribs are not for climbers! Be careful about putting toys into a toddler's crib; if he steps on top of them, it may give him just the boost he needs to make it up the side and over the bars. A fall from such a great height poses the risk of injury.

Some little monkeys surprise their parents by managing to climb out not long after their first birthday. Put some padding on the floor beneath the crib to soften it in the event of a fall. As soon as your little one begins scaling the bars, it's time to move up to a toddler bed.

Toddler beds are a significant next step because they have raised sides to keep youngsters from falling out—and from feeling afraid, they might fall out. They are also lower to the floor and pose less danger if a child finds it fun to climb over the side.

Many children are in love with their toddler bed initially because they're so easy to climb out of! Parents must decide whether it's better to lower the bars, which makes climbing less dangerous, or to keep the bars up to prevent a fall while sleeping. Another option is to have the child sleep on the mattress on the floor.

Since many toddler beds use the same size mattress as a crib, it's best to stick with the old one if at all possible. The familiar feel and smell of the old mattress can help smooth the transition from the crib. The quality of toddler bed frames varies dramatically from brand to brand. If you plan to lie down with your child to read stories or sleep, be sure to get a model sturdy enough to support both of you.

# Making The Transition

How will your toddler handle the transition from crib to a toddler bed? There's simply no way to predict it. It's smooth as silk for some, decidedly tricky for others. If a child is very resistant to change, slow to adapt to new situations, or a sentimentalist, leaving the crib's safety and security can be trying. Given a toddler's love of predictability and routine, it's a bad idea to let him step into his room to find his beloved crib gone. He may not see his parent's idea of a great surprise to be so fantastic. Perhaps he didn't like his crib at all.

Nevertheless, it was the steady friend that kept him safe night after night for as long as he can remember. If possible, provide a gradual transition. The secret to getting youngsters to give up their crib more willingly, many parents say, is to have them participate in the process from the very beginning.

# Staying Put

The toddler who won't stay put in a toddler bed poses a real dilemma for parents: What to do with a little one who hurries out of bed the minute parents have finished tucking him in? What to do with the bit of insomniac who rises in the middle of the night and forays into the living room when everyone is asleep? The first step to getting a child to stay in bed is to discuss it.

As with anything you are trying to teach your toddler, bedtime procedures are established with baby steps. Be patient and consistent as you train your child to stay in bed for the night.

Explain that it is dangerous for him to be up by himself, that he must stay in bed unless it's an emergency, and that he is to call Mommy or Daddy from his bedroom if he needs something. After that explanation, which a child may or may not understand, make it a policy to avoid further conversation studiously. Limit verbal exchanges to repeating in a firm tone of voice, "You're supposed to stay in bed unless it's an emergency. Go back to bed and call if you need something." (This assumes the parent has a baby monitor or is close enough to his room to hear him call.)

Walk him back to his room, help him a bed, issue another reminder to call if he needs something, and leave. Toddlers in this situation are apt to cry or get before you make it through the bedroom door. If that happens, turn around and go right back to his bedside to check on him, just as you promised.

In getting across any new idea to a toddler, you need to go one step at a time and show him how things are supposed to go. Stepping out of the room and turning right back around to go back in demonstrates what is to happen: He calls; you respond. That can provide reassurance that having to be a big boy sleeping in a big bed doesn't mean he is expected to be independent. If a toddler doesn't start climbing back out of bed the moment the parent turns to leave, that should be considered a victory.

It may seem inhumane to install a door protector and close the door to contain a toddler who keeps popping out of a toddler bed after everyone else is asleep. But given the danger youngsters can get into roaming the house, it may be the only recourse. Be sure to childproof the bedroom first completely!

Remain calm and matter-of-fact as you approach your child's bed, and say, "I heard you calling. Is everything all right? What do you want?" Provide a drink of water if a child says he's thirsty; do the monster check again if he's scared; then pat him and tell him he's doing fine, that it will take a while to get used to the new bed. Repeat the procedure several times, trying to avoid all conversation except:

I heard your call. What do you want?

You're okay now. It's time to get some sleep.

Good night.

Begin extending the time between visits to the child's room. Difficulty with the transition to a strange bed is understandable, too. Many adults have a hard time sleeping when they're away from home for the very same reason.

# Winding Down

Insisting that toddler's nap or go to bed when they aren't sleepy can provoke power struggles. Instead, have them observe quiet time. A noisy environment can certainly interfere with a child's ability to fall asleep. After entering dreamland, some can tolerate a lot of commotions; others remain susceptible to being awakened by sounds, especially during lighter phases of sleep. If you can't produce a quiet environment on cue, classical music can help to mask telltale sounds that suggest interesting happenings are going on elsewhere in the house.

To create a quiet and relaxing transition, help them unwind by providing soothing entertainment such as listening to music or looking at books. Bath time routines help, too. Discourage continued requests to get up by putting a kitchen timer in their bedroom. Tell them that, unless it's an emergency, they must wait until the alarm sounds before getting up or calling to you.

Once they do relax, sleep may not be far behind. Even if the rest doesn't follow immediately, children need to learn to relax and spend time entertaining themselves. Common strategies parents use to help their toddlers fall asleep include rocking them to sleep, singing lullabies, telling stories, giving back rubs, holding their hand, and taking the child into their bed.

Nursing and giving children a bottle to help them fall asleep is not a good idea, dentists say, because the milk pools in their mouth, rotting their teeth. The same problem applies to juice and other sweet beverages. Remember, only water!

Meanwhile, some desperate parents have gone so far as to childproof their little night owl's bedroom, leaving no outlet uncovered, no hard edge exposed. They empty it of all toys except board books, stuffed animals, and other toys that can be safely enjoyed without supervision, and remove all furniture but the bed. They install a gate across the doorway to contain their toddler and allow them to play until they're ready to sleep, instructing them to call Mommy and Daddy if they need anything. Then they head off to dreamland and let their night owl entertain herself.

# Exercise

Exercise relieves pent-up energy born of stress, tension, and the fundamental need to be on the go. Be sure your child gets lots of chances to run and jump and engage in active physical play during the day. A child's exercise class may encourage more sedentary types to move more and sit less. Then, spend more time engaging in quiet, pleasurable activities before naps and bedtime to soothe frazzled nerves. Try an extra-long bath, a second storybook, or a third chorus of a lullaby. Remember, however, that although stress can make it harder to relax enough to sleep, this too is something children need to learn to do. Anytime they can recover from an upset during the day, point it out. This skill will serve them well at night.

# Sleep Time Rituals

Rituals that induce relaxation can help toddlers make the transition from a busy, active day to sleep. Going through an invariable progression from taking a bath, hearing a story, listening to a lullaby, and saying prayers helps toddler insomniacs, just like their adult counterparts. As people come to associate the ritual with sleep, their bodies automatically begin to relax.

Many parents don't consider instituting naptime rituals, but they can make a real difference. It's good to communicate with your babysitters or child care workers, if possible, so that the routine never varies. Rituals should be designed to soothe, so avoid stimulating activities like roughhousing, tickling, and exciting or scary stories.

Some children engage in troublesome rituals such as repetitive rocking, which can escalate into headbanging, as a way to soothe themselves. It usually stops for eighteen months. You can help by not overreacting, by padding the sides of the crib, and by beefing up other bedtime rituals to provide a more gradual transition.

# Sleep Skills

The downside of all that rocking and singing and back rubbing and music playing to quiet fretful children and help them fall asleep is that they come to depend on someone or something outside of themselves—a real problem if they wake up in the middle of the night. Children need to learn eventually to handle the task of falling asleep—and of falling back asleep—unassisted.

# Learning to Be Alone

The first step is for children to learn to spend time alone. Being comfortable spending time alone in a crib or toddler bed is a prerequisite for falling asleep and for falling back asleep. By handing toddlers, a stuffed animal after they awaken in the morning or from a nap, leaving the room, and waiting five to fifteen minutes to rescue them, parents can give them time to practice being by themselves. Some experts say this can serve them well at night.

# How To Foster Identity

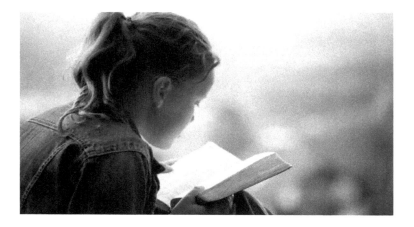

When dealing with strong-willed children, one of the issues parents struggle to overcome is their children's strive for identity.

Strong-willed children tend to fight for their identity just that bit harder.

One of the great advice I can give any parent is this "your child is not you."

Yes, we are parents, and we have a responsibility to help shape choices, but that doesn't mean we should make all the major decisions for them.

Allowing children to make their own decisions is crucial in them shaping their future character and identity.

I have talked to many parents who treat their children as miniature versions of themselves, whose sole purpose in the universe is to re-live their failed lives and fantasies. I have seen parents whose worldview has clouded their objectivity.

The adage is "the father's prayer is that his sons should be greater than he." We remember Albert Einstein, Bill Gates, and Isaac Newton. But does anyone remember who their parents were?

The point is that very often, children learn from their parents and often surpass their parents in many ways, and every loving parent should wish this should be the case.

The world is continually changing, and the rules are constantly changing, too, so we should guide our children and instill the values in them that will allow them to continue to be successful in the world they find themselves long after they fly the nest.

Regardless of how noble and lofty our ambitions are for our children, we must realize that our role is not to carve out their destiny but to help them create a life that will bring them fulfillment.

As parents, we need to be careful not to kill our children's creativity and individuality, especially if they are passionate about things we do not understand.

One thing is for sure, a strong-willed child is very stubborn about their passion and identity, and you must learn how to foster their development rather than destroying it.

Children may develop different dominant character traits. Some are introverts, while some are extroverts. Some children are confident, while others are shy and lacking in confidence. Some children are hard-working, and some are lazy and unmotivated.

Regardless of the dominant character traits, we must allow them to freedom of finding their own identities without being over-bearing.

If you are confident naturally and your child does not exhibit the same traits, do not make them feel something is wrong with them because they are shy. The best way to deal with features we do not like is to create an environment for development that does not make the child feel judged or below our expectations. Our job is to create a forum in which they can express themselves to their nuclear family.

A self-confident child will feel free to express their feelings about something. However, when the child has low self-esteem, they often become withdrawn and do not open up about what is bothering them. Parents can foster expression and individuality in children by being supportive. But first, they have to understand their children for who they are. Parents need to recognize their children's uniqueness and not try to force them to what they are not. Both internal and external forces can affect a child's personality. The parent must offer guidance to the child so that the child can make his/her own choices without feeling pressured.

How to foster individuality in a child?

When children are still young, they try to mimic your behavior in learning what the appropriate action is. The child's world slowly grows, and soon they start mimicking other children's behavior. When they join the school, they realize that they are part of a larger group. They try to find out how they can "fit in." You can guide your children into being unique in their way.

Here are some strategies that parents can use when they want their children to have better behavior in finding themselves.

# Understand Your Child's Perspective

When your child imitates another child's behavior, it isn't a bad thing. In so doing, they adjust their behavior. You can try to find out why they mimic that person. There has to be something that makes them desire to be like them. Maybe there are some other children that your child doesn't like, so he would try to adjust his behavior to differentiate himself from them. Other children want to get the same reaction that the other child gets. It could be the words that they use that make people laugh.

# Prevent Peer Pressure

Children who are not comfortable doing their things can quickly become vulnerable to peer pressure. That is why a parent needs to urge their child to be comfortable doing something. Since many people spend a lot of time in groups in school, they try to conform so that they can dress, speak, or act like the other members of the group.

These groups can be very influential in changing a person's lifestyle. Some groups can influence hairstyle, hair color, piercings in different parts of the body, tattoos, sexual relations, etc. They find comfort in such groups and would like to maintain their relationship, no matter what. If you let your child know that being different is okay, they will not be under pressure to do other things that they feel uncomfortable doing, to please their friends. When your child draws, dances, sings, or does any other activity, let them know that it is okay even if they do it differently from how others do it. However, this doesn't mean that you should teach your child not to have friends. Let your child know that despite the differences, they can still find common ground with friends.

## Share Your Opinions With Your Child

Connect and communicate with your child and let them know what you feel about certain things concerning his/her behavior. For instance, if your child has picked up bad behavior from his/her friends, emphasize the importance of good conduct. If your child starts using an inappropriate word that he/she heard from the friend, explain to your child why this word is wrong and why he/she shouldn't use it anymore. Your child will have reason to believe that you are right. When your child imitates, she is just experimenting. It doesn't mean that they will always be followers. As long as you show them some guidance, they will more likely choose good role models to emulate.

# Make An Impression

When your child isn't in school, you can monitor whom he/she spends time with that influences their behavior. It doesn't have to be someone. It could be something. If any children you feel can be an excellent example to your child, schedule a play date with your child. You want them to interact so that they can learn from each other about a thing or two. You should also engage in family activities, which foster good core values. It could be about giving back to society, volunteering, etc. your child can learn how to treat others by observing and listening to how you treat other people. Therefore, you should be a good role model so that your child can emulate these positive things.

# How You Can Encourage Your Child's Individuality

Let them have a say in what they wear. Let them develop their style by allowing them to pick what they can put on. If the child is too young, you can select two pieces of clothes and ask your child to choose one.

You should not dwell so much on what your neighbors are saying. This may prompt you to change the character of your child forcefully.

Please encourage your child to explore their identity.

Even if he/she takes some strange direction, it is still okay. At least, they are thinking about something unique for themselves.

Accept your children for who they are. What is meant to be will be? It would be best if you did not have a setup plan for your child's future. For instance, when your child is young, don't fixate your mind into believing that your child will be a doctor. Please don't force your child into taking a direction that they are not interested in. Let their interests guide them. As they grow, you can give them some pieces of advice, but you shouldn't force them to be what they are not or do not want. Celebrate their achievements in whichever field.

Take note of your child's likes, interests, talents, preferences, and attributes. It can help you in guiding them to do that which their heart desires. Please encourage your child to go after their dreams. Let them know that they can make it. Listen to your child so that you can learn about their aspirations.

Accept that the two of you are different, and you may have other likes or dislikes. Do not force your child to like what you like. Your child may dislike the things that you want. Know that your child is a unique being and not an extension of you.

# Do Not Make Comparisons Between Your Child And Others.

Do not compare him/her to yourself. Siblings can be very different. Do not reach them. This will create sibling rivalry, which can get nasty at times. It also breeds jealousy and hatred between siblings. Your child may begin to feel that he/she is not good enough, especially if you keep saying how the other sibling is far much better in many ways.

Examine how you are attached to their interests, appearance, and goals. How do you want your child to look or to present herself/himself to the public? Are you okay with it? Are you embarrassed by their choices?

# Encourage Your Child To Explore New Things.

When they are excited about an activity that they are part of, like the drama club, school choir, cheerleading, etc., they share in their excitement and be supportive. Attend their performances and encourage them to keep going.

# Emotional Factors Affecting Behavior

A child's sense of perception and reasoning is keen, but at the same time, it is fragile and easily impressionable. Just like physical factors such as sleep, hunger, and physical exertion, can cause unfavorable behavior changes, so can emotional or psychological factors. Things that can scar, hurt, frighten, or threaten a child's sensibilities are bound to leave lasting impressions on the child's behavior. Children have attack and defense mechanisms to counter what they consider a threat or overcome what scares them. We shall look at a few such things that are the most common factors observed that can change a child's conduct.

## Insult and Fear

Kids have a very delicate sense of self-respect and honor. A ridiculing comment, even by a well-meaning parent, about a child's work of art, for example, can seriously hurt a child. Cases of kids feeling insulted and humiliated so much that it affects their behavior are seen more in kindergarteners or kids of any school age. Kids starting preschool or kindergarten are exposed to different kids from various households, causing kids to defy around them emotionally. If the accompanying kids do not feel like threats, these defenses might well dissolve. But, insulting talk, laughter at each other's expense can often cause such kids to strengthen their emotional walls. These can very well carry back to the child's own home. Suppose they cannot communicate or unwilling to disclose what happened at school or the park to upset their disposition. In that case, this frustration and sense of humiliation will stay bottled up. This can cause kids to develop an inferiority complex and a deficient level of self-worth.

This was just one factor of feeling insulted. Perhaps, a different side of the same coin is fear. Feeling threatened by situations, intimidating adults, or even bullying school mates, can severely scar a child's innocent mind. This particular factor is more wide-ranged, seeing as a child can feel scared or threatened by many things. A menacing-looking man at a grocery store, a ferocious dog at a park or in a neighbor's yard, can considerably frighten a young mind, making a child feel threatened.

One of the most common consequences of feeling either scared or insulted is seeing a downturn in a child's health. The two most common ailments that young children suffer from are an upset stomach or the common cold with cough. There is a noticeable relation between these ailments and kids undergoing some traumatic experience, either a humiliation (for cases of a stomach ache) or fear of some kind (for insistent bouts of cold and cough). It stands to reason then that we don't just have emotional sensibilities and the resulting behavioral changes but also our kids' very health when faced with emotionally stressful situations.

All kids are different, and their reactions to different situations are equally as diverse. How one kid reacts to a threat might be entirely different from how another child would respond. What might be a situation of utter panic and fear for one could be a chance to prove themselves and step on the other's offensive? Their innate temperaments, mental constitutions, their environment at home, and interactions within the family, and their observations and inferences of the world around them will add to how kids would potentially react to stressful situations. An only child, or a first-born, or a highly pampered, overly protected, and doted-upon child, will undoubtedly be scared, feeling lonely, and exposed when confronting an intimidating scenario. Whereas, a child who has seen brothers and sisters fight, seen their siblings come back from school after an argument, or any such other exposure, would be at least a bit better prepared for any unpleasant situation outside of their homes.

Withdrawing oneself in a shell, going quiet and inexpressive, being secretive about even simple day to day activities are only a few possible changes observed in a child feeling scared or bullied. A decrease in self-worth, low self-confidence, and a strong sense of inferiority can be seen in a child who is always made fun of, even if the joke is small. If it happens enough, it has the potential to scar a child's confidence permanently.

# What Can We Do?

Talk about it. We can and must talk even before we see signs of emotional stress in our kids, but more so if we see such signs. Establishing a trusting and friendly relationship with your child is essential. Your child must not hesitate to come to you and relieve their emotional burdens at your feet when they face a problem. It would help if you were their first choice of a confidant. Are you there at the top of the list of their best friends? If not, there is a need for you to work on your trust-acquiring skills. Whether your child is facing bullying at school or constantly insulting jibes from a mean cousin, you must become the first person your child turns to. Talking is your tool to gain their trust. Talk with them to lift their spirits, to restore their confidence, and to help them see themselves in a better light.

Make sure to keep your comments and observations genuine. Fake praises and false encouragement would cause more harm than benefit. It would hurt their self-respect more to find that your words and talk weren't honest. For those kids who are struggling with fear, you must talk to them to gain their faith to share their worries with you. It would help if you were a pillar of strength and security for them. Please take steps to ensure their fears are taken care of. Enquire into situations or about persons that scare them and work toward addressing the issue. If they can witness you standing up for them and removing things that scare them, it will strengthen your bond. And this is always a good thing.

## Wishes and Wants

Unfulfilled emotional needs and desires are the most significant factors to affect a child's behavior. These are extensive parameters with a broad scope of what can fall in between. From basic and vital needs to the most trivial and silly wishes, kids can get affected by them. Depending on age, such unfulfilled needs can cause slight to severe changes in their behavior in kids. For kids, things like needing a hug, wanting a new toy, or a pat on the back, are all personal wishes and wants even though their path to fulfillment is physical.

One must tread carefully when dealing with a child's emotions. An adult might not understand the significance of wanting to go to the park, ice cream at an ungodly hour or take the dog out for a walk in the middle of the night. What seems silly, laughable, and downright humorous for an adult can be a huge deal in a child's eyes. Children can quickly become stubborn, unreasonable, and throw one tantrum after another if their wishes aren't fulfilled. So how do we understand what the child needs, why it's important to them, and how to fulfill or deny their want in a harmless way?

While dealing with a stubborn child wishing for something impossible, it is essential to keep the child's age in mind and remember the three age groups and our supposed focus for each of them. For kids under three, your attention, love, and care in the world for them. There is hardly room for rules or discipline. For kids of this age group, you must deal with the utmost love and care in handling their wishes. Try diverting their minds to more plausible options for entertainment or games, or some such distraction far off the subject. Though these wishes can cause displays of stubborn behavior, there are chances of far more permanent effects of such unfulfilled desires. Improper handling can cause kids to develop spite toward the adults dealing with them. Many older kids have also been known to turn revengeful when their wishes aren't met. All this can be avoided and resolved by using the right technique while handling a tantrum.

Kids live in a constant stream of observing, learning, and adopting scenarios. It is reasonable to understand that when a four-year-old watches his younger brother playing with a toy and wishing he had this toy, he feels within is a mixture of jealousy, anger, and resentment. Mild reflections of all these emotions, for someone so young, but they are there. You deny your child extra TV time, and he throws the cushion across the hall; what he is feeling is anger. Kids do not know what these emotions are called. There is always a new emotion for them that comes to the fore in different situations. If you can establish a connection with your child early on, then you can help him calm these new emotions and experiences and get him to label them appropriately.

One might argue as to how naming emotions could benefit kids. For one thing, your kid's emotional range is expanded, and he or she can acknowledge it, and more importantly, a child recognizes the emotions to stay away from along with being able to identify these emotions when present in others. It helps them decide which emotions are safe to hold on to and explore, and which ones are to be rid of for maintaining a healthy mind. It contributes to the overall growth of the child as a sensitively alert person.

# Curiosity Of Your Toddler

"Curiosity killed the cat."

If I could say one thing to my son, that would be it. He is very interested in many things. He is eager to explore and try out new things without realizing the dangers of his uninhibited exploration.

Children's curiosity to learn motivates them to try new things and find out how it works. It is an innate quality of a child, and it drives them to step out of the boundaries you set for them.

A child's curiosity can be a double edge sword. Children learn by exploring the environment around them. I was clueless with my firstborn, so here are some tips of what to expect when your child's curiosity has been piqued:

- Imitating Mommy. My son became interested in everything that I was doing. Doing the dishes, washing clothes, cooking meals. He would imitate my actions like when he would try to slice his food with a spoon or pour his drink on his bib, trying to wash it.

- I want to see inside. This drove me crazy as he tried to open every drawer in the cabinet and pulled everything out, scattering them all over the floor. He is not looking for anything in particular, mind you; he wants to see what is inside.

- Wet and Wild. Oh, this one was the pits. The first time I found him playing in the toilet bowl, I could not stop screaming. He was playing with the water, throwing his toys one by one to see if it will float or sink. It is not just the toilet bowl, sometimes the fishbowl, the garden hose, and the bathtub. He loves playing with the water period.

- Play, hide, and seek. I had to fill every nook and cranny in the house to keep him from crawling inside. He would crawl in small spaces, hiding and waiting for me to find him. He fell asleep in one corner, and I almost tore the house apart looking for him.

- Play Jack and Jill. You got it. He climbs on every furniture he could reach and climb on. He even tried climbing the stairs and called out to me in the middle of the stairway. I do not remember how I get him so fast, but I did. I hugged him and held him so tight while crying. My husband found us sitting at the bottom of the stairs with me, still crying.

These are just a few samples of my son's idea of exploration. I knew his curiosity stems from wanting to find out more about things and the world around him.

I have no problem with him wanting to explore, but I have a big issue regarding his safety. I noticed my son's curiosity had increased his growth in many ways.

- An increase in his physical growth. My son's skill improved with the addition of his physical activities. There is visible growth in his eye and hand coordination, as he can now move objects and place them in the right place.

- Intellectual growth. Asking questions gave him answers that lead to another question. I know it can be exasperating at times, but he discovers new things and understands how it works. With the help of his five senses, he can determine the taste and smell of food. He can differentiate sour from sweet.

- Social and Emotional Growth. Exploring taught my son that there are other children like him outside of the home. He also knows that Mommy is always there to talk to him and guide him, making him feel more secure.

Seeing his rapid growth encourage me to help nurture my son's growing curiosity. There was no need for me to push him to be curious because it seemed innate in him. I need to make sure that his burning curiosity will not die down.

## Developing His Curiosity

There are many ways to nurture your child's curiosity, but here is what worked for me:

- Learning from his cue. Find out what your child's interests are. Do not push ideas to him. Allow him to raise ideas of his own.

My son showed interest in anything on the water. He loves watching our aquarium as the fishes' swim by. When he started asking me if he could breathe in water just like the fishes, I would admit to getting alarmed because he might test the idea. I explained to him the difference between fishes to humans. I started bit by bit, allowing him to do follow-up questions to know he understands me and not bogged down by information.

- Answer their questions. Do not try to evade or give vague answers to their problems because it hinders their development. Give them answers that would provide them with the opportunity to ask another question. If you do not know the answer, tell them straight and tell them the two of you can try finding solutions. A quest can be thrilling to a child. However, remember that your response to a two-year-old may differ from how you answer a 12-year-old.

My son, one day, asked me if he could swim in the water like the fish. When I replied yes, he asked me how. I explained that he needed to learn how to swim first. It did not end there, he followed it up with some more questions, and it ended with me promising to teach him how to swim like a fish.

- Let them read. Books are windows to another world. Let them explore the new world by reading books. It does not matter if their interest is in comic books. As long as it captures their imagination, it will pave the way for exploring new ideas.

To encourage my son's interest in underwater creatures, I bought him books about aquatic animals. I also purchased a giant aquarium to house other underwater creatures. Together, we set up the new aquarium and named each fish inside.

- Create a stimulating environment. Make their room and your house as enjoyable as possible. The images and shapes they see around them will open up their imagination.

Aside from the aquarium, I bought glow in the dark underwater creatures and decorated his room. I also added photos of water sceneries like falls, rivers around the house to allow his imagination to soar.

My son's interest was not just in underwater creatures. He had other parts too that I learned to cultivate. I still worry always about his safety, but I can address the issue by ensuring that my son will always be in childproof places. Accidents happen, and you cannot control it, but you can lessen its chances by putting safety measures.

What is essential is to allow your child to explore and learn. Let their imagination soar.

Yehuda Berg once stated, "As youngsters, our minds are lively, and our hearts are open. We accept that the miscreant consistently loses and that the tooth fairy sneaks into our rooms around evening time to put cash under our cushion. Everything astonishes us, and we think the sky is the limit. We constantly experience existence with a feeling of novelty and unbridled interest."

# CONCLUSION

*Thank you for reading all this book!*

**Montessori Knowledge**

From the moment they enter the school, the Montessori procedure promotes order, coordination, focus, and independence in the children. The student's emergent self-regulation — the ability to teach oneself and think about what one learns from young people to young people — is promoted by school design, materials, and everyday routines. The sequence of Montessori lessons harmonizes well, often exceeding the standards of state learning. That way, children are presented with complex learning concepts through practical experiences that lead to profound knowledge.

The Montessori curriculum is deliberately grouped into three-year cycles instead of divided into annual student learning expectations. This is because children develop and master academic topics at different speeds, and children often work in specific fields in spurts. The instructor supports the progress of the child in all aspects of the curriculum to ensure that he or she is introduced to the full series of lessons in each area to provide encouragement and challenge as appropriate.

*You have already taken a step towards your improvement.*
**Best wishes!**

CPSIA information can be obtained
at www.ICGtesting.com
Printed in the USA
LVHW020957050521
686547LV00010B/878